Well-earned praise for
The Diet Docs' Guide to Permanent Weight-Loss...

"Dr. Joe is truly an innovator in the field of nutrition experts."

JIM CORDOVA, MR. UNIVERSE AND PRO WORLD CHAMPION BODYBUILDER

"People all over the world come to me seeking diet advice, but when I have a question, I go to Dr. Joe!"

DAVE GOODIN, UNIVERSE, INTERNATIONAL,
AND WORLD CHAMPION TITLES HOLDER

"I have been able to far surpass my goals only because of Dr. Joe's expertise and encouragement."

MICHELLE SHEPHERD,
PRO WORLD FIGURE AND FIT BODY CHAMPION

"With remarkable candor and unexpected humor, *The Diet Docs* deliver what America needs to know: the truth...Using a common-sense approach based on extensive personal and professional experience, Scott and Joe educate readers on the science of nutrition and provide the all-important psychological support to make your change to a healthy diet a *permanent* part of your life."

MICHAEL R. HARRISON, M.D., FELLOW AMERICAN COLLEGE OF
CARDIOLOGY (FACC), PRESIDENT, EVANSVILLE HEART CENTER,
VOLUNTEER CLINICAL ASSOCIATE PROFESSOR OF MEDICINE,
INDIANA UNIVERSITY SCHOOL OF MEDICINE

"Scripture instructs us to honor God with our bodies. That is not an easy mandate to follow in our..."super-size me" culture. But with *The Diet Docs' Guide to Permanent Weight Loss*, Drs. Joe and Scott provide a time-tested nutritional plan to lose and keep off the extra pounds. You won't find a fad diet here—just solid nutritional information packaged for the average joe!"

PASTOR JEFF HUDSON, DIRECTOR OF MATURITY,
CHRISTIAN FELLOWSHIP CHURCH

"We use the Diet Docs' book as an education reference for our Family Medicine residents. It provides a realistic template for practicing family physicians to help their obese patients achieve a safe and sustainable weight loss."

K.A. VOLZ, M.D., DIRECTOR,
DEACONESS FAMILY MEDICINE RESIDENCY

THE DIET DOCS'®
GUIDE TO
PERMANENT WEIGHT LOSS

Joe Klemczewski, PhD   J. Scott Uloth, PhD

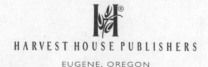

HARVEST HOUSE PUBLISHERS

EUGENE, OREGON

All Scripture quotations are taken from the HOLY BIBLE, NEW INTERNATIONAL VERSION®. NIV®. Copyright © 1973, 1978, 1984 by the International Bible Society. Used by permission of Zondervan. All rights reserved.

Front and Backcover author photos © Todd Burnett

Cover by Left Coast Design, Portland, Oregon

Readers are advised to consult with their physicians or other medical practitioner before implementing the suggestions that follow. This book is not intended to take the place of sound professional medical advice or to treat specific maladies. Neither the authors nor the publisher assumes any liability for possible adverse consequences as a result of the information contained herein.

THE DIET DOCS'® GUIDE TO PERMANENT WEIGHT LOSS
Copyright © 2008 by The Diet Docs, LLC
Published by Harvest House Publishers
Eugene, Oregon 97402
www.harvesthousepublishers.com

Library of Congress Cataloging-in-Publication Data
Klemczewski, Joe.
    The diet docs' guide to permanent weight loss / Joe Klemczewski and J. Scott Uloth.
        p. cm.
    Includes bibliographical references.
    ISBN 978-0-7369-2465-8 (pbk.)
    1. Reducing diets. I. Uloth, J. Scott. II. Title.
    RM222.2.K568 2008
    613.2'5—dc22
                                                                        2008020669

Printed in the United States of America

08 09 10 11 12 13 14 15 16 / BP-KB / 10 9 8 7 6 5 4 3 2 1

Contents

Scott's Story 7

1. First Things First 17

2. Carbohydrates—Not Just for Breakfast Anymore 27

3. The Skinny on Fat 45

4. Power to the Proteins 61

5. The Diet Docs' Rx 69

6. Meals, Power Spacing, & Other Fun Stuff 93

7. Use It or Lose It!.............................. 105

8. The Psychology of Success 121

9. Your First 6 Weeks 129

10. Great Health Benefits! 145

11. Pitfalls and Obstacles 165

12. Keeping Excess Weight Off Forever............... 193

13. Food Prep & Recipes 199

    A Diet Doc Five Years Later 261

    Bibliography 263

Scott's Story

J ust how in the world did I get here?" The flashing red lights blinked between my toes as I asked that question over and over. I was 229½ pounds! The perfect weight—if I were a 6'2" linebacker for the Colts. However I'm 5'8" (5'7¾" as my wife is quick to remind me), and I have the 40-yard dash speed of a 3-legged turtle. That last half-pound taunts me, and I chastise myself for buying a digital scale. I'm closing in on my fortieth birthday and I'm 60 to 70 pounds overweight. How on earth did this happen?

I'm sure this scene from my life is repeated multiple times a day in bathrooms and locker rooms around the world: people staring at scales and wondering how they went from svelte, healthy kids of the past to the overweight, chronically sick, and fatigued adults of the present. Those blinking red numbers are warning lights of impending doom.

The next disaster film from Hollywood shouldn't feature a wayward comet, global warming, or icebergs. No, it should be our swelling abdomens and poor health brought on by lack of proper nutrition, lack of exercise, and our woeful lack of information. ("Captain, the 32-ounce soda cup is about to crash into the Atlantic and give everyone on the Eastern seaboard diabetes. What shall we do?") Scares me—does it scare you?

According to the PBS documentary *Diet Wars*, 50 percent of America's children will become afflicted with diabetes and all its complications. Obesity may soon replace smoking as the single largest preventable cause of death in the United States. What we need to avert this disaster is practical information that we can realistically incorporate into our daily lives. We need a weight-control process that's attainable and sustainable.

My weight problems started almost immediately after high school. I believed I needed sugar and caffeine to stay conscious in college, so Mr. Mountain Dew and I were tight. Then when I stopped running cross-country to focus on my studies my girth expanded. Furthermore, there was the never-ending supply of fattening food at the student union where I would eat a bowl of Captain Crunch for dessert after a huge meal. My "freshman 5" quickly turned into the "freshman 15." It deteriorated from there. I rationalized my behavior by believing I was simply sacrificing my health in pursuit of knowledge, a good job, and helping others. That seemed like a decent trade at the time.

Like many, I labored under the delusion common to former athletes: I could "turn it on" and instantly return to the 155 pounds I was when I graduated from high school. Needless to say, by my senior year of college I'd gained 40 pounds. As I was soon planning to marry my high school sweetheart, I started bike riding, lifting weights, and playing basketball to shed those extra pounds. I eventually managed to work off 20 pounds and was down to 175 by my wedding day. I was proud of myself and didn't think I looked half bad.

But it didn't last.

The next four years of medical school and three years of residency solidified my soda addiction…and my rationalization skills. My medical education improved my knowledge of nutrition to a certain extent. The application part was the problem.

Then, in the Lamaze class my wife and I attended the husbands had to wear a padded "sympathy belly." I joked I didn't need one since I already looked nine months pregnant. Frankly, the number of people who patted my stomach and asked me when I was due was more than a little annoying. I knew I would never shop in the "tall" section, but having to purchase suits in the "big" section was really bumming me out.

I wish I could say my nightmare on the scale was enough to stop me, but it was easier to quit weighing myself.

How many of us delude ourselves into believing we'll be "just fine"? How many of us procrastinate going to doctors because we're scared of what they might find? How many of us believe we need to make a serious life change but don't have the necessary information—or perhaps the will—to succeed? How many of us live in fear that we can't do anything about weight and health anyway, no matter how hard we try? And how many of us are stuck in habits we think we can't break? ("Gotta have that soft drink in the morning or I can't start my day.")

If that sounds familiar, I have news for you: I was right there with you. I believed all those lies. I thought I was doomed to be "fat and happy." Even though I had a doctorate-level education in medicine, I still didn't have the right information to help myself. I knew I needed assistance…and that's where this book comes in.

I'm blessed to live in the same community as "Dr. Joe." I'd witnessed the amazing transformation of several people who attended our church who had been helped by Dr. Joe. These people lost weight, looked wonderful, and were bragging about how great their energy levels were. So I bit my lip, sat on my ego, and took action.

Joe has built a career combining academic learning with real-world education. He has a degree in physical therapy and two doctorates, including one in health and physical education. He's also a professional bodybuilder with arms that make Popeye look like a slacker. Joe knows what he's talking about.

After a year and a half of working on my own to get in shape, I felt I had conquered the exercise demon through my regular treadmill routine and I lost a few pounds. However, when it came to nutrition, I definitely needed more information. I also needed to learn the importance of supplementing my exercise routine with weights.

When I stood on Joe's doorstep, I was stalled at 213.5 pounds. After consulting with him, I learned more about nutrition than I'd learned in my first semester of medical school. He is truly the Sergeant Joe Friday of nutritionists. This book is the "just the facts" culmination of our knowledge about effective (and permanent) weight loss.

The key thing is that Joe and I are not just health or medical gurus. We're just a couple of hard-working, regular joes (well, one regular Joe and one slightly irregular Scott), who both continue to actively practice in our respective fields. Our goal is to help you arrive at that moment of true understanding about yourself that will change your life forever. That moment when the lightbulb comes on. When you say "Aha!" and are able to get the simple principles that will help you lose weight, be much healthier than you are now, and enjoy your life more fully.

People are often swept away by the murkiness of the science of nutrition. However, nutrition is a "hard science" with testable end points. In this book we show you how to reach those end points in an easy-to-understand fashion.

Some people want to be told "eat this" or "don't eat that"…which this book can do to a point. But that kind of legalism won't forge a lasting change in behavior. Only with *understanding* will you develop a habit of healthy eating that can last a lifetime. We want to be your partners to help you achieve that goal.

There is no magic or voodoo available or necessary to make those unwanted inches melt away. It's science—but it ain't rocket science. In fact the basic tenets of weight loss as we describe in this book are exceedingly simple…once you're armed with the necessary knowledge of how your body metabolizes food and the motivation to make some changes in the way you live.

With a few rare medical exceptions, there is absolutely no reason any person can't lose weight if he or she follows the guidelines in these pages. I wish I had a nickel for all the people who came into my office blaming a thyroid disorder for causing them to be overweight, only to sit there the next week with their lab tests showing their blood chemistry was perfectly normal.

Throughout these pages you'll learn the value of your own personal "macronutrient range," which we'll refer to as *The Diet Docs' Rx*. This critical range of macronutrients keeps you losing weight without making your body think it's starving and slowing down your metabolism.

The Diet Docs' Rx chart in chapter 5 provides the proper amounts of protein, carbohydrates, and fat for men and women based on height. You will learn how to glean nutritional information right from the food labels without having to use a calculator. You will also discover why portion sizes are so critical to success.

As my ten-year-old daughter, Gracie, says, "We're not on a diet; we're on a healthy eating plan!" This plan restricts calories by tailoring protein, carbohydrates, and fat to the levels that will fit your body structure and type without overutilizing any one of the nutrients.

You will benefit from the clinical application of this diet that has helped others combat diabetes, coronary artery disease, hyperlipidemia, and osteoarthritis. Finally you will learn from someone who lost more than 60 pounds—me!—what it was like and how you too can lose the unnecessary weight you now carry around. We stress nutrition, exercise, discipline, and the fun that leads to permanent weight loss and ultimately good health.

The place to start is to come to that moment of truth when you stop making excuses. I'm a physician who works 60 to 80 hours per week. My day used to consist of arriving at the hospital by 7:00 a.m., doing rounds checking on my patients, and then going to the office and seeing patients all day (and usually taking only 10 to 15 minutes for lunch). I was so busy I didn't even feel I had time to go to the bathroom.

I would get home between 6:30 and 7:00, eat dinner, play with my three children, help get them ready for bed, and start doing paperwork at 9:00. I usually finished between 11:00 and midnight.

Rise and repeat, day after day. I had developed extraordinary discipline in my business life, but chaos ruled my eating habits. "Anything, anytime, anywhere" was my mantra. Maybe I just wanted one aspect of my life that I didn't have to care about—at least not now anyway.

When could I find time to exercise? When could I find the time to eat right? I had to be mentally sharp. I needed those three sodas a day. I'm a big boy, and I chose this life and how I'm going to live… or mis-live…it.

Then one day I realized I could fall over dead and some people would simply step over my corpse and say, "Oh, poor Dr. Uloth. He was such a nice man. I wish he'd taken better care of himself. I wonder who else in town is taking new patients?" It doesn't matter what your job is or how important you think you might be. At some point it's game over, man. Game over.

The truth is, no one else will get you healthy for you. Not your mama, your daddy, or your spouse. You have to decide, like Morgan Freeman asked in *The Shawshank Redemption*, are you going to "get busy living or get busy dying"?

I came to understand that as long as I was still vertical I wasn't going down without a fight, especially when I thought about the people who loved me. I knew God tells us to treat our bodies like a temple— and my temple was in utter disrepair. I had a T-shirt that said "God's property" on it, and one of my friends quipped, "If that's God's property it ought to be condemned!"

I realized then that I was robbing my wife and setting a shameful example for my patients and, more importantly, my children. I realized that doctors should be helping patients *prevent* disease instead of just treating it.

Trust me: It's a darn sight better to be eating in moderation outside of the hospital than sipping your dinner through a straw in the post-op recovery room. Good health is serious business, folks, and for that reason, this book is serious about offering you the path to a better life. That path, although narrower than what you're used to, is a lot more fun to run down with your family than struggling down the wide path of abuse in agony.

At the time of this writing, I have gone from 230 to 169.5 pounds (44 pounds lost with Joe in 6 months as opposed to the 16 I lost in 18 months on my own). I'm currently past my original goal of 172 pounds—the weight that's considered healthy for my height. Nowadays I'm actually glad I have a scale that weighs in half-pound intervals!

I recently bought a pair of 34-inch pants and took my 42s to the Salvation Army. I have run my first consecutive mile since high school. Do I have six-pack abs yet? Nope and I probably never will, but I can see a little definition in my abs rather than my belly obscuring my toes when I look down. So instead of "abs of steel," I'll be happy with healthy abs of aluminum foil.

In family medicine, if you need to consult on a tough problem, you call in a specialist. When it comes to weight-loss and good health, Joe is that specialist. He helped me understand that I didn't have to lose all my excess weight in 90 days or some other unrealistic time frame. He pointed out that it took years to build up that weight and that it would take 6 to 12 months or more to get the weight off and to tone up my muscles so I would achieve the results I wanted.

The nutrition information Joe gave me is not overly rigid—and it worked within my schedule. It provides the flexibility of my personal macronutritional range and takes into account what I want to eat... within reason.

I also came to realize that I could get up early and exercise, and I don't have to lift weights three or four days a week (two days are fine) to get stronger and help burn unwanted fat.

I came to the point of being satisfied ordering salmon and veggies with no butter instead of a cheeseburger and fries. Actually, it's *more* satisfying because I've gained a mental victory and real progress toward my goal. Not only did I enjoy the change in *what* I ate, but also in *how* I ate. By eating three meals and two snacks a day, I found that my blood sugar became much more balanced. I now have greater energy. And since this program is more moderate in carbs (unlike some other rigid anti-carb plans), I have the mental sharpness I need.

Carbohydrates are necessary to power the brain and nervous system, whereas ketones (the byproducts of an ultra-low carb diet) have a terrible time crossing the blood–brain barrier. That's why you may feel like a walking zombie on low-carb diets—headachy and lethargic.

I now have no caffeine during the week and have gone from three Mountain Dews a day to one on Friday (as a reward for making it through the week). Understand that even the most disciplined athlete needs rest. Part of The Diet Docs' Plan includes one "splurge meal" a week. You don't have to deprive yourself 24/7.

Another benefit I noticed: In the past when I was plagued with various ailments, I always attributed them to my constant exposure to illness in my practice. However, these past few years I've been healthy and strong—obviously more resistant to diseases and infections. I believe this has been a result of The Diet Docs' plan.

So is it any wonder I've jumped at the chance to work with Dr. Joe to help others learn to live happier, healthier lives? Joe often says there are two types of clients who come into his office: one who is determined to do anything it takes to achieve his or her goals and one who is constantly looking to cut corners and see what he or she can get away with. This book has the information you need to succeed. However, you have to decide if you're going to be the first type of client or the second. Self-control is where it starts.

Ultimately, having a good and healthy body isn't about triumphing over the bully kicking sand in your face at the beach. And it sure isn't about the next high school reunion reality show. This is real life. Health and happiness are the goals.

You spent your hard-earned money for this book, and we sincerely hope you take the time and energy to follow the plan. We've written it in terms we think you'll be able to grasp easily. And we've arranged it with the expectation that you will want to return for refresher readings in the future.

We believe that after just a few weeks of results you'll realize the decision to get healthy was worth it. Joe and I are here to support you. You will succeed! And not just for today, but for a lifetime. Don't be intimidated. Get busy living!

Transformation of a Diet Doc

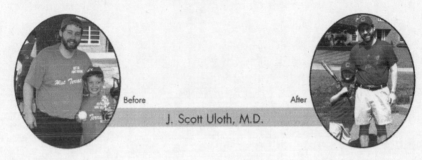

Before   After

J. Scott Uloth, M.D.

First Things First

If you've purchased this book, chances are you've also purchased other diet books in the past. You're probably hoping this one offers a final workable solution to your attempts at weight loss.

It does.

The Diet Docs' plan is simple, scientifically sound, and it works. It's straightforward in that it can be explained in just a sentence: To lose weight, you must help your body burn the excess fat it's been adding and storing while you've been eating improperly (and probably not getting the exercise you need).

It's scientific because it takes into account how your body—and all human bodies—work. You'll learn how to help your body work with you to shed that excess weight for good.

As for its workability, if Scott's opening pages didn't convince you, we're going to scatter some other testimonies throughout the book from people just like you who have successfully lost weight using the The Diet Docs' Rx for permanent weight loss. Their stories make it clear that you too can succeed.

Although the plan is simple, its effectiveness depends on three keys vital to success.

1. *Learn to eat the right foods to help your body burn the stored weight.* In order to learn to eat the right foods, you need a basic understanding of the three all-important "macronutrients" you consume daily. These macronutrients are the basic fuels your body uses in various combinations to survive and thrive. They also determine whether you gain, lose, or maintain weight. The macronutrients are protein, carbohydrates (carbs), and fat.

Macronutrients are counted in grams per serving and are listed on the side of most packaged food and drinks (except most alcohol). If you haven't already developed the habit of reading food labels, you will need to do so. Pay particular attention to serving size. Are the values listed for five nuggets or six? This may not seem like much, but that's a 20 percent difference! Even what you think would be an obvious serving size may actually be two servings or even two and a half. Drinks, especially soda, are notorious for that. A 20-ounce bottle is 2.5 8-ounce servings, so if you drink it all, you have to multiply the carbs and calories by 2.5. Knowing the value of what you put into your body is crucially important. On The Diet Docs' Rx you will be keeping track of the amounts of the three macronutrients you consume daily. Don't overlook this critical step.

Chapters 2–4 examine these all important macronutrients in detail.

2. *Adding appropriate exercise to further boost weight loss.* Any successful weight-loss plan must include some form of repeated physical activity. The multiple health benefits of exercise—beyond weight loss—don't need to be debated here. From a clinical perspective we can tell you that most fit elderly patients have "taken some exercise" for decades. We have some 70- and 80-year-olds who can do many energetic push-ups.

True, it's *possible* to lose weight without exercise (good nutrition takes care of that), and to someone who is gravely obese or disabled, that may be where you'll have to start. However, for the majority of us who *are* able to exercise, it's crucial that we move. Chapter 7 will help you get moving.

3. *Staying motivated.* Learning about macronutrients is perhaps the easiest part of the weight-loss process. Even incorporating some exercise into your life may be harder than this third element: *becoming and staying motivated for the changes that must happen if weight is to be shed and kept off.* Success in permanent weight loss can ultimately be traced to a person's willingness to change. Weight loss is not as easy as some of the infomercials make it sound.

An important part of staying motivated is having realistic expectations. People are built differently. I, Scott, will never, ever have arms like Joe's, even if I lift weights until I'm 80. However, Joe will never be as tall as I am. Ha! But the fact that you're not blessed with a certain physique shouldn't stop you from going to the gym and working out. Don't waste your life agonizing over your supposed flaws. Even the "beautiful people" constantly want someone else's lips, buns, or chest. God's Word says you are "fearfully and wonderfully made," so accept your genetic makeup and work on the best you that you can be. This is about *your* transformation.

The Diet Docs' plan will give you some shortcuts and the information you need to achieve weight loss *and* a higher level of fitness. But just like the proverbial swampland in Florida, always beware of diet plans that sound too good to be true. Any diet that tells you that you won't have to watch what you eat or exercise to achieve your goals is a complete lie. Have you ever really known anyone who successfully "burned calories while they slept"? Give me a break. Those programs are deceptive and lead to despair among the dieters who try them. Our plan is based on scientific facts. It can help you turn your life around if you are dedicated to changing your bad habits. And you *can* do it! You are stronger than you think you are.

See Your Physician

Speaking of the physical aspect of weight loss, as you begin to implement The Diet Docs' plan, you'll want to let your doctor know. We suggest you have a physical checkup. We're not just putting this in to give the lawyers something to do; this is a critical part of your total health. Many health problems are not outwardly visible. High blood pressure, thyroid problems, early propensity to develop dia-betes, and many other potentially dangerous conditions are best de-tected early.

We know many people don't want to go to their physicians be-cause they don't want to be lectured on their poor health habits. I, Scott, didn't see my physician for a couple of years because *I* didn't want to hear what I knew he'd say either. We all prefer to camp out by that river in Egypt: De Nile. It's nestled right next to the crumbling ruins of the food pyramid.

Just remember, your doctor is your partner, not your parent. You need to be monitored and to have someone in your corner during your commitment to permanent change. If you discover you have a problem, you and your doctor can work together to defeat it rather than being pulled under the water of De Nile by one of those currents of hypertension, diabetes, or coronary artery disease. To those of you who have already discussed your weight issues with your doctor and wouldn't miss a yearly physical, great job!

While seeing your doctor, do *not* ask for diet drugs to jump-start your weight loss. You don't need them. You will likely lose five to seven pounds in the first week. Medications are not without side effects (check with the Phen/Fen people), and you can only take them for a certain period of time by law. Time and again we see people take diet drugs, lose a few pounds, and one year later they're back to their previ-ous weight and asking for more drugs. Even gastric bypass, which is a life-changing operation, has its risks. But on The Diet Docs' plan, we've seen people lose 100 pounds or more without resorting to some-thing as drastic as surgery. It's much better to apply the principles in these pages, lose five to seven pounds in the first week and one to two pounds a week thereafter. It may not be quick, but it's the healthy, sensible way to lose weight. Plus it won't harm your metabolism, which will make it easier to keep the weight off for good.

If you need a friend or a loved one for support in the days ahead as you implement the plan, ask them. However—and this is very important—it is your responsibility to lose weight and no one else's.

Unless you need support, you don't need to tell your friends, neighbors, or cat you're going on a diet. You don't really need someone to hold you accountable. The only one you would cheat is yourself. Let's face it, "food eaten in secret is delicious" (Proverbs 9:17). Solomon understood that 3,000 years ago—and the Thighmaster hadn't even been invented yet!

Let me say it again: The only one who holds you accountable is you. Not your parents, your spouse, your friends, your coworkers. You can nibble that cheesecake when your accountability partner isn't there, but the calories still count. And you haven't fooled anyone. You'll then step on the scale and wonder, *Why isn't this diet working?*

Hmmm, I wonder why.

Preparing for Battle

Now, some basic information to get you started.

- First, read this book all the way through. That should be fairly obvious, but we have known plenty of people who have abandoned a diet book because it was too complicated or too boring. Hopefully this book is neither and can be read leisurely in a weekend. Only a complete understanding of the principles taught will allow you to apply these strategies effectively.

- Buy a digital food scale of decent quality. Some people say that having a food scale is a bit obsessive, but can you accurately tell what four ounces of meat looks like or how much one ounce of nuts is? People will use the "size of a fist" or the "size of a deck of cards" comparison, and that is helpful in a pinch, but we have seen people make their fist small or the size of the Incredible Hulk's, depending on how hungry they are. If you're going to develop healthy eating habits, it's critical to weigh your food when you can, especially in the early phases of your diet.

Some may have discovered after weighing their meals that they often underestimate the amount of food consumed by 50 to 150 percent! Take the guesswork out of the picture. Be precise. Estimating rather than weighing may not make a lot of difference if you're eating tuna, but it could mean the difference of 10 versus 20 grams of fat if you're eating red meat.

Serving size has been so distorted by restaurant entrées that weighing is a good way to get things back into perspective and achieve a true and healthy portion size. Don't want to take a scale to work? Then don't. Weigh the food in the morning or evening or on the weekends. After a while you'll have a much easier time correctly estimating portion sizes of the foods you eat regularly.

• Purchase proper measuring cups. (For the culinary impaired, there is a difference between measuring cups for solids and liquids.) Scott was very naïve about cooking (Hamburger Helper, Dinty Moore Beef Stew, and spaghetti were all he managed in college) and didn't realize that one fluid ounce does not equal one ounce by weight, no matter how many times his eighth-grade home economics teacher told him the difference. One cup of a dry cereal by volume does not equal eight ounces by weight. There are usually only 14 ounces in an entire box.

Scott's former breakfast routine seemed healthy, but upon closer examination it was just the opposite. He would pour orange juice in a travel mug, grab a breakfast bar, and head out the door to work. He thought he had about 8 ounces of liquid, but when actually measured, it was 12 ounces. Then when he read the label and found out how much sugar is in juice, combined with the high number of carbs in the breakfast bar, it wasn't hard to figure out why his weight loss was so slow. That little science experiment only took a few minutes to calculate, but it taught him a valuable lesson.

- Get a journal. The kind doesn't matter. You just have to be faithful to write down whatever goes into your mouth. A truism in medicine: Document everything. This is not obsessive. It's a semi-objective way to see where you might be having problems. Develop the discipline of writing food down. Those little candy bar miniatures add up when you eat several a day. The difference in 200 carbs versus 125 is very substantial over time (That's 300 calories per day!). Also a journal is useful for keeping track of your exercise and giving encouragement to yourself. You don't have to buy an expensive notebook. I usually get a devotional journal that has blank pages and jot down columns for protein, carbs, and fat. I add them up as the day goes on.

- Unless you're good at adding in your head, get an inexpensive calculator. You'll be totaling your amounts of three macronutrients (protein, carbohydrates, and fat). Keep it simple.

- Get a food-count or values book. These usually are sold in the diet section of your local bookstore. A food count book shows the true nutritional values for many foods. If you're not sure about the value of a certain food, and you know it may have a lot of fat and carbs, be careful. Take only a small portion.

- As for a scale...to weigh or not to weigh your body, that's the question. Whether 'tis nobler to watch thy downward progress or to wail at the upward slide of the needle...we don't have a good answer to that one, folks. We've already talked about Scott's love/hate relationship with his scale, but he hasn't thrown it out the window yet.

A scale can be a good tool to learn what foods affect you and what you can do to combat the upward slide. For example, some people learn they are more sensitive to fat calories than carbs. If they overdo it on fat intake, they would gain weight. It would also take much longer to lose than if they overate a little on their carbs. Scott liked to weigh daily initially because it helped inspire him and encouraged his new healthy habits (walk, weigh, hit the showers, prepare for a day of healthy eating). When you weigh, use the same scale at the same time of the day. Wear the same amount of clothing. Most people find that a salty meal during the evening will show up on the scale the next morning. Women will find their weight increasing due to water retention during their monthly cycle. Whatever you do regarding the scale, keep going. Don't be discouraged. If you're consistent, the weight will come off.

Some people foolishly allow their scales to control their moods, which goes up and down, fluctuating regularly. If you can't handle the truth and a "bad scale day" sends you into the "I suck so I'll just eat an entire pan of brownies" state of mind, don't weigh daily or don't weigh at all. To thine own self be true. Know yourself and your limitations. The scale is simply a tool. It's not a mechanical judge of your worth.

Okay….you have an appointment with your doctor, you've made a shopping list for the items mentioned, and you're getting motivated, right? Great!

Key Points

1. The Diet Docs' plan is based on solid science.

2. Be an active participant in your success.

3. No one is the same metabolically or personally. While providing the right structure, The Diet Docs' Rx allows maximum flexibility.

4. See your physician for a physical—you're overdue.

5. Take responsibility, be consistent, track your food, and educate yourself. You are now on your way to becoming your own nutritionist!

The Diet Docs in Action...

Audra's Story

I was always active, which worked great with my passion for horses. They're a lot of work! I competed in equestrian events and operated an equine breeding program that involved daily horse care, putting up hay, and handling feed. Like most of us over our busy adult lives, I gained a few extra pounds. I didn't get too shook up about it since I could still out-work the teenage boys in the hay field.

After major surgery my doctor suggested that I lose the extra 40 to 50 pounds since I wasn't getting any younger. After explaining I wasn't the Twinkie-popping couch potato he pictured, I told him that when I attempted to watch my diet, I ran out of energy when completing my farm chores and tending to my full time job. He handed me a piece of paper with a phone number and told me I would benefit from nutritional counseling. My first reaction was, "What? I always grab a glass of orange juice and a banana on my way out the door each morning! What in the world could be wrong with that? It's not a doughnut, for crying out loud!"

Little did I know! Everything was wrong with it. Reluctantly I called and soon met with one of Dr. Joe's associates. I bought Dr. Joe's book and headed home. As I sat down to read, I thought, *How is this one any different from all the others in my bookcase?* But it *was* different. For the first time in my life I understood what was wrong with my breakfast, along with all the other convenience foods I consumed on a daily basis.

My first trip to the grocery store for shopping Dr. Joe's way took me more than three and a half hours. Talk about a field trip! I'm sure security was watching and asking, "What in the world is this woman up to? Is she planning a robbery, stalking someone, or just plain crazy?" I stuck to the plan and the weight started falling off. It was amazing!

Unfortunately I wasn't mentally or emotionally prepared for the turn of events that soon unfolded in my life. I would soon know the frustration felt by Wile E. Coyote every time he blew himself up, got smashed by a boulder, or ran off a cliff. Along with an unplanned career change and stressful personal events, the next five years were plagued with numerous injuries, which included a patella alignment surgery on my left knee, a dislocated right knee from being kicked by a horse, a fractured right arm and leg after being run over by a galloping three-year-old filly (no quarterback has ever been sacked like that!), and injuries from a defective air bag exploding when I started my car. If I were a horse, they would have shot me!

continued —➤

My bout of depression turned self-destructive, and I gained back the lost weight and then some. Toward the end of 2006 I turned 39, weighed 302 pounds, experienced constant knee pain, and my physical activity was nonexistent. I realized something had to change, but how? Luckily I saw Dr. Joe's ad in a local paper and remembered the book that was still in my bookcase (and a little dusty). And hey, didn't my family doctor, Scott Uloth, do the diet and help write a new edition? He seemed pretty enthused about the project. I read the book again and decided to give it a try once more, but I didn't tell a soul in case I failed. Just like before, the weight started falling off. I had to ask, *What went wrong before? Why did I quit when my life turned upside down?* I pondered this for weeks until I saw another of Dr. Joe's ads, and this answer hit like a ton of bricks: support.

That was the help I needed. It still took me a few days to gain the courage to make the phone call that would change my life forever. Dr. Joe met with me, addressed concerns regarding my injuries, and provided the inspiration and motivation I so desperately needed. Dr. Uloth attented one of the lectures I was at and kept emphasizing the key points of the diet when I met with him in his office.

I have lost 118 pounds and am within 35 pounds of my goal weight. I am lifting weights twice a week and doing cardio training. I have reduced my knee pain to almost nonexistent and am back in the saddle again! Thanks to The Diet Docs, I will be living the rest of my life instead of merely existing.

The other day I went on a cruise with my son and father. When we went before, all I did was gorge on the buffets. This time I was zip-lining across treetops! Living, not existing; experiencing unbridled passion and freedom.

If you had the opportunity of a lifetime to do something as dangerous as climb Mt. Everest, would you take that risky adventure without a guide? Of course not! So don't even think of embarking on this life-changing journey without The Diet Docs. Guys, "thank you" will never be enough for guiding me to my summit and beyond.

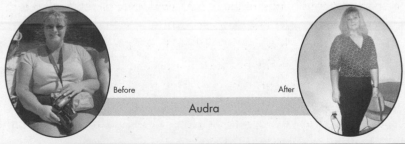

Before   After

Audra

CHAPTER 2

Carbohydrates–
Not Just for Breakfast
Anymore

Food is divided into three main "macronutrients": carbohydrates, protein, and fat. Each form is dramatically different in structure and function.

A calorie is a unit or measurement of energy. One gram of carbohydrate equals four calories. The same for one gram of protein. Fat, often called a more dense nutrient, has nine calories per gram. Even though each calorie is the same unit of energy, the effect on your body's chemistry and function is quite different depending on its source (protein, carbs, or fat). That's why some methods of weight loss are more effective than others.

Identifying the macronutrients and how they work in your body is the cornerstone to the nutritional aspect of The Diet Docs' Rx, which is the core of this diet plan. Due to their importance, each macronutrient will be covered in its own chapter: fat in chapter 3, protein in chapter 4, and in this chapter we'll discuss the most controversial—carbohydrates (carbs).

Friend or Foe?

Many dietitians and nutritionists have elevated carbohydrates to an almost untouchable level of nutritional deity. For decades diet gurus devised weight-loss schemes where eating carbohydrates were at the center of the plans. Until recently commercials bragged about how cereals were full of "nutritious carbohydrates." (Now the catch-phrase is "whole grains" since the low-carb craze has made "carbo-hydrate" a dirty word. They don't mention that processed white flour isn't a whole grain.)

Long before nutrition was a studied science, it was understood that athletes needed more fuel—more calories—to support their training. As is true now, carbohydrates were the most abundant, least expensive, most convenient, and usually best-tasting food. Since athletes were observed consuming many more carbohydrates than anyone else—and had physiques that were admired by all, the conclusion was drawn that eating carbs was the way to go.

What most people didn't realize was that most athletes eat a

Average Joe Physiology

Double Your Fat Loss

In a review of isocaloric diet studies (diets that compare the same amount of calories but with different ratios of protein, carbohydrates, and fat), it is difficult to find outcomes different than was found by the *International Journal of Obesity*. Some studies were of people consuming 1,000 calories and divided into higher-carbohydrate/low-fat groups and higher-fat/low-carbohydrate groups. Other studies were reviewed using the same type of nutrient ratios but even higher calories. The groups on lower carbohydrates but the same amount of overall calories lost 43 percent more weight. That is a strong indictment against high-carb diets, but it's not necessarily an endorsement of low-carb diets. Carbs have their place and going to extremes in eliminating or consuming them will cause major problems. Carbohydrates are a key diet variable, but the correct level to consume depends on several factors, which we'll discuss.

great deal of carbohydrates and don't gain body fat only because of their intense levels of training. But that's not so for nonathletes who don't work out as hard. And just because athletes may get away with eating an abundance of carbs because of their energy expenditure, does that mean it's the best nutrition even for them?

The inevitable response to one extreme is the opposite extreme, so it didn't take long for low-carbohydrate diets to creep onto the scene like a brain fog.

So what's the truth concerning carbs? To find out, let's turn to metabolic physiology. Once you understand exactly what happens inside your body when you eat different foods, you'll be able to better discern good nutrition from bad.

Carbohydrate Structure and Function

Carbohydrates provide most of the energy for our bodies most of the time. Because they require the least amount of work for the body to break down, carbohydrates are the easiest of the macronutrients to digest and be converted to glucose. Carb sources are loosely described as sugars, starches, and fibers, and are commonly known as simple and complex. We typically think of simple carbohydrates as junk food, such as soda and candy, and complex carbs as whole foods, such as potatoes, pasta, and bread. But this type of categorization leads to the false assumption that a particular food is either good or bad when actually it should be seen more on a continuum. Worst, bad, good, better, and best are more appropriate ways of describing carb choices. This will become clearer as you understand how they compare to one another and how they affect your body.

Glucose is the smallest sugar molecule possible. It's the form of sugar that the human body uses for energy. Whatever form of carbohydrate you consume, the end result of digestion is glucose. There are many forms of carbohydrates, and the process of digestion that leads to glucose is what can affect your energy level, mental acuity, physical functioning, and even athletic performance.

You may recognize the names of various forms of sugar: glucose, lactose, fructose, maltose, dextrose, sucrose, and so on. Each one of these carbohydrates has a different level of molecular complexity. Those that are made primarily of glucose are easy and quick to digest since most of the carbs are already in the smallest possible form (for dieters, that's bad). Those with a more complex molecular structure are harder to digest and take longer to move through the digestion process (that's good!). The *Glycemic Index* (Figure 2.5) is a scale that ranks carbohydrate foods by comparing their structures. It reveals the simplicity or complexity of the carbohydrate source.

Two Rebel Carbohydrate Sources

Two caveats that need explanation are fiber and sugar alcohols. The popularity of low-carb diets has led people to believe that fiber and sugar alcohol are "free" and don't need to be counted. Fiber, though it *is* digested slower, is still a carbohydrate. Fiber not digested in the stomach may be broken down in the large intestine. So while fibrous carbs are good, healthy sources, they are still, and must be counted as, carbohydrates.

An interesting carbohydrate source that the FDA hasn't classified firmly is sugar alcohol or polyphenols. Used in some baked products and very prevalent in protein/energy bars, sugar alcohol (usually in the form of glycerine or glycerol) is actually part of a fat molecule.

Being calorically similar to a carbohydrate but structurally coming from a fat molecule, and the fact that it's digested very slowly without a fast rise in blood sugar, originally led the FDA to not require it to be listed on food labels. Talk about denial! We don't know what it is, so we'll just ignore it? We don't think so! Whether due to lobbying efforts by low-carb food producers or due to the reduced danger to diabetics (since it doesn't cause a fast rise in blood sugar), sugar alcohol was allowed to fly under the radar.

When the outcry was finally loud enough, the FDA started requiring both fiber and sugar alcohols to be rightly listed in "total carbohydrates" on the label, but they continue to allow fiber and polyphenols to be deducted to create a new category: "net carbs." But these carbs are present in your food and need to be counted. So don't deduct fiber and sugar alcohol from your totals. Ignore the confusing net carb counts and track only your *total* carbohydrates.

Alcoholic beverages are similar but don't even (as of yet) bear the "net carb" label. Look at any low-carb light beer and you'll find near zero protein and fat counts, a low carbohydrate count, and calories listed at a much higher level than if you did the math. (Remember: Protein and carbs have four calories per gram and fat has nine.) The "missing calories" are carbs not counted—sugar alcohol. Wine and hard liquor are roughly four grams of carbs per ounce, though they'll be often listed as just one. Light beers are really 20 to 25 grams of carbs, not 7 to 10 as many people think.

Carb Basics

When you consume a high-glycemic index carbohydrate such as white bread, a banana, a baked potato, soda, or candy, you're consuming a carbohydrate that's primarily glucose. Little digestion needs to take place. They pass through the stomach quickly and enter the small intestine. Absorption occurs in the small intestine, and since so much glucose enters so fast, uptake is rapid. Your brain closely monitors your blood sugar levels, and such a rapid increase triggers your pancreas to release the hormone insulin. Insulin is the storage hormone that shuttles blood glucose to where it's needed.

Most of us aren't glycogen-depleted (short of stored glucose), so our muscles and livers usually contain *plenty* of glucose for fuel. Depending on how many carbohydrates you consume at one time, chances are you will have too much blood sugar and nowhere to store it. Your already high level of circulating insulin causes your liver to convert the blood sugar into triglycerides (fat) to be stored. Insulin also triggers body-fat cells to pull excess glucose in to be converted directly into body fat.

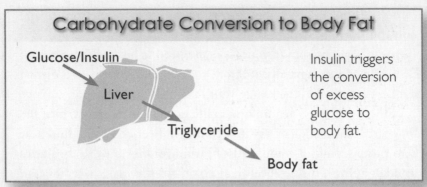

Figure 2.1

None of the high-glycemic carb sources I just mentioned have fat in them, but a large portion of the carbs can be converted to fat due to the effect of insulin. Unfortunately, the problems don't stop there. By storage, utilization, or fat conversion, your blood glucose levels return to normal and your brain tells your pancreas to stop releasing insulin. However, even with the process stopped, a certain amount of insulin remains active in the bloodstream until it is "used up." This means more blood sugar will be removed, dropping your blood sugar below the normal level. A blood sugar level too low makes you feel tired, as in the case of after-lunch dozing behind your desk. Even

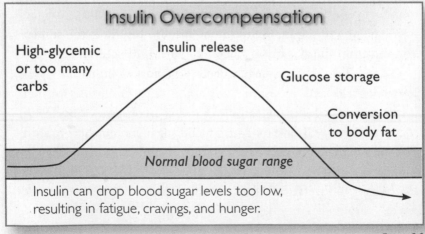

Figure 2.2

worse, your brain sends out powerful hormonal messengers to signal hunger. I'm sure you've experienced eating something and being even hungrier a short while later. Too much of a drop and you can have more severe symptoms such as hypoglycemia. That's why you might end up weak, shaky, and starving 30 to 60 minutes after eating.

The tragedy of this process is you go from bad to worse in body composition, energy level, and health in one fell swoop. You either block body fat loss or store new body fat with a "fat free" food. You then end up tired and so hungry with carbohydrate cravings that you eat a similar meal and start the process all over again. This is an extremely powerful biochemical reaction. Massive, seemingly uncontrollable binges are birthed by insulin-induced low blood sugar. Many of us live on this roller coaster and don't realize we're the ones causing it. We say, "I just have a slow metabolism" or "People naturally gain more body fat as we get older." You've used these excuses, and you probably believed them. It's time to gain control over your nutrition.

Falling Off the Wagon

Any one of us can overeat occasionally, but bingeing can become an eating disorder. Bingeing is often rooted in dieting too hard. When you sustain too low of a carbohydrate level for too long, your body is going to crave carbs, and most of us aren't going to be able to stop eating once we start. This is common but devastating. Here's an example in an e-mail from one of Joe's clients:

> So...I knew it wouldn't take long before you discovered the real me. I haven't sent you this week's food diary, but suffice it to say that it's not good at all. This is me. Unable to stick to clean eating for more than days at a time, disgusted with myself, and firmly believing that it is my destiny to be chubby and miserable all the time. Yet I make these choices. I understand that each time I eat ice cream or chocolate or whatever I'm making the choice to do so. What I don't know is why I can't seem to correct my behavior. And I

don't consider myself one of those people who cheats just to try to get away with as much as possible. No, I try. How I do try...then I crack and I eat something I shouldn't because I just HAVE to...then I can't stop so I eat more. Then I feel guilty and disgusted with myself. Then I get into a cycle of "Well, you've already screwed up so if you do it again it doesn't matter." And I do, which perpetuates the cycle. Then I get really mad at myself and say, "Okay, get over it, move on, you'll be okay." And I go great guns and do really well until yet again, after days of pacing around my kitchen looking at food or gazing at the giant cookies at the supermarket, I give in and the self-destruction begins again. "Well, I screwed up and ate the cookies so if I eat this cake too it doesn't matter." It doesn't seem to matter how much variation I get, how many carbs or how little, there is stuff I WANT and I can never seem to shake it. And it's very bad when I'm at work with all the treats people bring in. I know my choices only hurt my chances of achieving my goal, yet I do it anyway. Through weeks and weeks of dieting I tell myself how much I'm sacrificing and suffering and I think, *Why go through all of this and then mess it up for a piece of pie?* But somehow I manage (in the moment) to justify that it won't matter. Am I insane? Am I just a loser?

Have you been here? We have. Scott would say that if he didn't drink any soda he would be fine, but if he had even one before the end of the day, it would turn into three or more.

There are three critical points to see in that e-mail. The first is the cycle. If you don't give yourself a chance to move away from the dominance of over-consuming carbohydrates, and if you never get past that "sticking point" and make it into a couple days of stability, you may stay in that miserable cycle.

The second point is that it does take a few days for your body to stabilize, and it *does* get easier. Hunger decreases, cravings decrease— a very noticeable shift.

Both of these points are physical. It's sugar withdrawal, and you have to get through it. These biological impulses are going to happen regardless of how strong- or weak-willed you may be in the moment of temptation. Power spacing, which is covered in chapter 6, will help you get through this detox.

The last point is your will. During those tough points, it helps to develop a sense of righteous indignation: "I'm not putting *that* into my body!" Or a sense of mission and pride: "Being lean means more to me than that cookie! I can do it!" Avoid having tempting foods around and ask those around you to help. Do anything you think will help, but get beyond this roller coaster and eating right will be easier. Once you move into a deeper level of body fat metabolism through controlled and consistent carbohydrate intake, stability will be just around the corner.

Stability Can Be Controlled—by You!

The goal in The Diet Docs' plan is control thereby bringing nutritional stability to your body. So by understanding the physiological problems created by eating too much or too little (getting too high and spiking your insulin, thereby causing fat storage, or getting too low and setting off a hypoglycemic eating binge) you'll be better equipped to gain *permanent* control.

When you must have a treat, don't view yourself as a failure. Everyone loves a treat. Simply learn to make better choices for that special snack. Eat in control, keep close to your ranges, and you'll be fine. Quit putting yourself in a shame spiral and beating yourself up. You *can* stay in control!

Caution: Don't let sugary treats become a habit and replace a large portion of your carbohydrate allowance. You might be able to fit 46 grams of carbs from a soda into your daily range, but you'll be crowding out healthy carb sources, such as fruits, vegetables, and whole grains, in addition to harming your pancreas and making your body work harder to lose weight. Concentrate on health and the things that will help you succeed.

More Complex Carbs

What if you chose a carbohydrate on the other end of the glycemic index, such as a grapefruit, an apple, a bowl of oatmeal, or even a salad? These carb sources have different molecular configurations of glucose. Fructose, cellulose, galactose, and so on are much more complex forms of carbohydrate. When these hit your stomach, digestion takes longer to break them into usable glucose molecules. Since this process takes more time, the molecules enter the small intestine and are absorbed more gradually. Blood sugar levels rise slowly, avoiding your body signaling for a major insulin increase.

By changing the carb source, you've decreased the potential for the creation of new body fat! And your energy level will rise over the next couple of hours instead of rising and plummeting quickly. Another plus—and possibly best of all—hunger is dramatically reduced because blood glucose levels are stable instead of too low.

During a particular new client consultation, Joe's new student said, "So keeping insulin low is the whole key?" Though there are so many swirling factors occurring at once and so many things depend on one another or affect each other, the answer was yes.

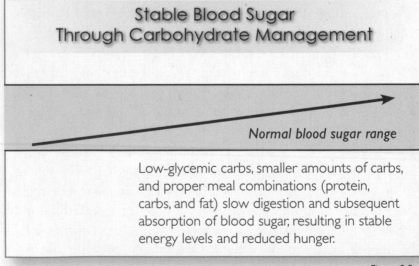

Stable Blood Sugar Through Carbohydrate Management

Normal blood sugar range

Low-glycemic carbs, smaller amounts of carbs, and proper meal combinations (protein, carbs, and fat) slow digestion and subsequent absorption of blood sugar, resulting in stable energy levels and reduced hunger.

Figure 2.3

Insulin and glucagon are the two opposing hormones that keep blood sugar either increasing or decreasing. If we need more glucose, glucagon is produced and through all the complex machinations discussed, we end up losing fat. When there is excess glucose, insulin is produced to bring blood sugar down. Part or most of the excess is stored as fat. We're either storing or retrieving. When carbs are eaten in smaller and appropriate amounts according to your personal Rx (discussed in chapter 5), insulin is held at bay and glucagon is present more often and in higher amounts. Voila! Body fat loss. An oversimplified explanation perhaps, but it is the whole key.

Work with Your Body

Glucagon 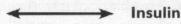 **Insulin**

Glucagon	Insulin
• Released when blood sugar is low	• Released when blood sugar too high
• Signals body fat cells to release triglycerides	• Signals body fat cells to convert glucose to fat
• Liver converts fat to glucose	• Signals liver/muscle to store glucose
• Blood/liver/muscle glucose/glycogen stabilizes	• Causes rebound blood sugar drop
• Hunger decreases	• Hunger increases
• Energy increases	• Energy decreases
• Metabolism increases if protein intake high enough (at least short-term)	

Figure 2.4

Meal Combinations

The glycemic index is extremely important to your dieting success. Some nutritionists don't place much value on this tool, and some act like it doesn't exist. Yet it can be your greatest asset or your fiercest enemy.

Many individuals have enjoyed early dieting success with fault-less nutrition and then unknowingly eaten a high-glycemic carb and were slammed with raging hunger and an insulin-induced tailspin. We've all been there. Four or five days into a diet, we find ourselves at the bottom of a gallon of ice cream or lying on the couch with our pants unsnapped after an extended visit to the all-you-can-eat buffet. Now that we know what causes that behavior, we won't let it happen again—right?

The same thing can occur, though, if we go too low on carbo-hydrates for too long. Anyone who has followed their peers over the low-carb diet cliff knows that powerful hormonal cravings are unleashed that even the strong-willed can't withstand. Both missteps lead to the same demise. A badly timed high-glycemic carb or going too long without carbohydrates can lead to low enough blood sugar levels that you will suffer from unnecessary hunger, an energy crash, or a head-first dive into a binge.

Your gastrointestinal system actually gives you a carbohydrate safety net, if you know how to use it properly. So far we've looked at examples of low- and high-glycemic carb digestive pathways. The glycemic index is a continuum; every food fits in somewhere.

Obviously staying in the low-glycemic index as much as possible will offer the best results with the least discomfort. But what if you *really* want a carb source that's not as low on the index as you wish it was? Protein and fat molecules are larger and denser than carbo-hydrates, and digesting them takes between one to three hours... and sometimes longer. If you eat a carb source in combination with fat and protein, the carbohydrate gets caught in the slowed down digestive process.

Stated another way, a carb eaten alone will be digested and absorbed much faster than one eaten with fat and protein. Slowed absorption of carbs is a very good thing! On the practical side of nu-trition, every meal or snack doesn't have to have a "perfect" balance

Sample Glycemic Index Selections

The glycemic index essentially rates the speed of digestion of carbohydrates and thus the impact on blood sugar elevation. A zero rating could indicate no carbohydrates present. Glucose is rated at a value of 100 and very simple carbohydrates can reach a value much higher than 100.

	Glycemic Index Value	Serving Size	Grams of Carbs per Serving
Cereals and Breads			
All Bran	30	1/2 cup	15
Oatmeal (rolled oats)	42	1/2 cup (dry)	27
Oatbran bread	47	1 slice	18
Rye bread	58	1 slice	14
Raisin Bran	61	1/2 cup	19
Pancakes	67	two 4"	58
Special K	69	1 cup	21
Bagel, white	72	1	70
Grape Nuts	75	1/4 cup	22
Shredded Wheat	75	1 cup	30
English muffin	77	1	14
Whole wheat bread	77	1 slice	12
White bread	80	1 slice	14
Crispix	87	1 cup	25
Rice Krispies	87	1 cup	21
Corn Flakes	92	1 cup	26
Snacks			
Potato chips	57	2 oz	18
Blueberry muffin	59	3.5 oz	47
Tortilla chips	63	2 oz	30
MET-Rx Bar	74	3.6 oz	50
Soda crackers	74	5	15
Rice cake	82	1	7
Pretzels	83	1 oz	20

Figure 2.5

	Glycemic Index Value	Serving Size	Grams of Carbs per Serving
Common "Starch" Sources for Meals			
Pasta, wheat	32	1 cup	32
Pasta, white	38	1 cup	32
Sweet potato	44	5 oz	25
Rice, brown	50	1/2 cup	17
Rice, long-grain	61	1/2 cup	18
Rice, white	87	1/2 cup	28
Potato, baked	85	5 oz	30
Fruit			
Cherries	22	1/2 cup	10
Grapefruit	25	1/2	11
Apple	38	4 oz	15
Pear	38	4 oz	11
Orange	42	4 oz	11
Peach	42	4 oz	11
Grapes	46	1 cup	24
Banana	52	4 oz	24
Raisins	64	1/2 cup	44
Cantaloupe	65	4 oz	6
Pineapple	66	4 oz	10
Watermelon	72	4 oz	6
Vegetables			
Broccoli	15	1 cup	5
Cauliflower	15	1 cup	5
Lettuce	15	1 cup	2
Carrots	47	1 cup	10
Peas	48	1/2 cup	10
Corn	60	1/2 cup	18

(We recommend *The New Glucose Revolution* by Jennie Brand-Miller for further values and a deeper understanding of the glycemic index.)

Figure 2.5 cont.

of nutrients, and sometimes you can eat a carbohydrate food alone. Between meals that contain good amounts of protein, once in a while a stand-alone carb is a great snack—especially something healthy and low-glycemic such as a piece of fruit or vegetables.

Carbs, Carbs Everywhere and Not a Drop to Eat

Now that all those nice Keebler elves have magically removed the nasty old trans-fats from their products, we should be safe, right? Unfortunately some of these types of foods are still crammed with carbs, and we're not talking the good kind.

"Good carbs" come from whole grains, fruits, and vegetables. Fiber is critically important to help slow carb absorption. It also helps bind cholesterol and limits its uptake. Think of fiber as a sponge that soaks up fat and pulls it out of your digestive pathway. That's why oatmeal boxes have those charming little red "Heart Healthy" logos on them. "Bad carbs" include processed white flour, sugar, high-fructose corn syrup (which is used as a sweetener in just about everything), and even a few fruits and vegetables.

We are hesitant to label a potato or banana as "bad," but they are much higher in carbs and are absorbed much faster than other produce. The key to remember is that faster absorption means more intense insulin spikes, which means a roller-coaster ride in emotions, food cravings, and health. Insulin is "bad" if you have too much of it circulating because of an overload of carbs. (Bad, hormone, bad! Back to the pancreas where you belong.)

We take in far too many carbs in our usual diet, and it's so easy to do. Slurp down a can of soda—a few minutes and there goes 35 to 50 carbs and up to 200 calories. Go to your favorite fast-food chain and you may consume more than 150 carbs in a single meal. (Yeah, you can have your big toys and your big burgers and then have your big heart attack and face big medical bills.)

The backlash against carbs had "experts" recommending eating much more of the other two macronutrients (protein and fat) and keeping carbs to an absolute minimum. However, there are a couple of problems with that logic. You are never really "cured" of your carb "addiction." Your body will always require a certain amount of carbs to power your central nervous system. You can never, ever be completely carb-free or your body will not function properly. You can certainly try to prevent yourself from bingeing on sugar, but you need a certain amount of glucose to power the organ that makes you human and holds all that useless sports and entertainment trivia.

Furthermore, lack of natural fruits, grains, and vegetables leads the "low-carbers" to frequently need fiber supplements. Most people aren't really interested in a diet that causes them to spend more time in the bathroom or hundreds of dollars in powdered tree bark. A supplement should be just that—a complement to an already healthy diet and lifestyle. Natural fiber is crucial for keeping weight down, and in our experience, people would much rather eat natural fiber than mix it up in a glass or take it in a pill. A study by Dr. Simin Liu showed that women who consumed more whole grains not only weighed less but also had a 49 percent lower risk for weight gain than those who had lower intake. (Now if people refuse to eat fiber in their diet, fiber supplements are better than no fiber or the use of laxatives.)

The Diet Docs' Rx helps limit calories by increasing lean protein to decrease hunger, followed by a moderate amount of healthy carbs and lower fat—a healthy diet you can follow your entire life. Everyone will have a different spin on how to decrease calories, but you want a diet *you* can stick with over time. A systematic review of the efficacy and safety of low-carbohydrate diets presented in the *Journal of the American Medical Association* in April of 2003 came to the following conclusion:

> There is insufficient evidence to make recommendations for or against the use of low-carbohydrate diets, particularly among participants older than age 50 years, for use longer than 90 days, or for diets of 20g/day or less of carbohydrates.

Among the published studies, participant weight loss while using low-carbohydrate diets was principally associated with decreased caloric intake and increased diet duration but not with reduced carbohydrate content.

Dang, those science geeks are long-winded! But they make a great point.

Key Points

1. Carbohydrates are your body's primary source of energy. Limiting carbohydrates forces the body to use an alternative energy source: body fat.

2. High-glycemic carbs promote body fat creation, increased hunger, and decreased energy.

3. Low-glycemic carbs increase energy, decrease hunger, and help to avoid body fat storage, as opposed to high-glycemic carbs.

4. Combining carbs with fat and protein slows absorption of carbohydrates (see chapter 6, "Meals, Power Spacing, and Other Fun Stuff").

The Diet Docs in Action...

Carl's Story

In June I visited my family doctor for my annual physical. I weighed almost 250 pounds, had high blood pressure, and a total cholesterol count around 215. The real story on the cholesterol was the triglyceride number. That is the actual fat that cruises through the bloodstream. Mine had been very high for several years, and the doctor had me on cholesterol-reducing medicine. Now he wanted me to start taking medicine to control my blood pressure.

I told the doctor that I'd been able to control my blood pressure in the past by losing a little weight. He said, "Lose the weight!"

Soon after this, I got an e-mail from a friend about his experience with Dr. Joe. Now, I'd been exercising regularly for several years. I did weight lifting at the gym and owned my own Aerodyne. But I decided to talk to Dr. Joe and was amazed at how easy the nutritional plan was. All I had to do was log what I ate and count protein, carbs, and fat to get the correct balance to metabolize the fat in my body. Exercise isn't enough. I read the book and started eating to live rather than living to eat. Basically that means only eating what is required for my body to do its work.

I immediately saw results in weight loss and realized I was losing the fat and not the muscle because my weight lifting was improving. In six months I lost over 50 pounds of fat and my muscle tone became obvious. My cholesterol is now in the low-normal range with no medication and my triglycerides are almost nonexistent. My blood pressure and pulse rate are in the very healthy range too. This is with nutrition control and no medication. Now my family doctor is recommending Dr. Joe to other patients.

I'm 49 years old and feel better than I did when I was 30. I enjoy myself at restaurants and don't worry too much on vacations. If I gain a few pounds I know how to lose the excess in days. It's all about being in control of what goes into my mouth. Dr. Joe is a great encourager and helped me realize that life is worth living to the fullest. I did it with nutrition control and reducing the medications. And you can too!

Before

After

Carl

CHAPTER 3

The Skinny on Fat

The Great Myth

Eat anything you want as long as you don't eat fat." Have you heard people say such a thing? This myth has been an accepted fact for a long time—until recently, that is. You will still find that idea printed in some nutrition textbooks, but we're at least two fad-diet generations beyond counting fat grams.

We've gone from removing every drop of fat from a chicken breast to eating bacon, burgers, and butter as part of the trendy "eat anything you want as long as it's not carbs" diets.

The popularity of low-carb diets (such as the Atkins Diet and the South Beach Diet) has started people thinking about what they eat. Most important, it has challenged the government and the food industry to address, in a research-based fashion, what healthy eating really is.

Carbs have become the mainstay of dieting, but this newfound nutritional enthusiasm has caused a spillover into taking a close look at our old nemesis, dietary fat.

A very positive step many food processors have taken is pulling trans-fats from their production process. The chemical alteration of these fats leads them to be far more harmful to our arteries. Partially hydrogenated soy, palm, and palm kernel oil used to be staples in snack foods, but now manufacturers proudly proclaim: "0 grams of trans-fats!" Thanks! It's about time!

People have instinctually and correctly believed that the natural dairy fat that's in butter and cheese, along with animal fat, is inherently better for them than any chemically altered product. Trans-fats are truly *not* "better living through chemistry."

Every family seems to have a story of a 90-year-old grandfather who ate bacon, sausage, and eggs every morning and cooked them all in lard. However, these folks of earlier generations lived lives of sun-up to sun-down labor that allowed them to burn many calories while improving their musculoskeletal and cardiovascular systems. Furthermore, they ate whole grains full of fiber that naturally helped decrease the body's ability to absorb cholesterol. Today we eat grains that have had all the fiber pounded and bleached out of them, and the only workout we get is the stick shift in the car or the Wii controller.

It's very clear that too much fat isn't good for us, and thinking we can indiscriminately consume any amount of fat as long as we keep our carbs low is not wise.

Although the American Heart Association and other organizations may not have gotten everything right with the emphasis on low-fat and higher-carb (let's not say "high carb" because we honestly don't believe that's what was ever advocated), it has been clearly shown in multiple studies that a diet too high in animal fat increases risks for stroke, heart attack, and certain types of cancer.

This does not apply to certain types of plant-based fats or fish oils that have been shown to be protective. A study in the *Archives of Internal Medicine* showed that one handful of mixed nuts can decrease the risk of coronary artery disease. Nuts have monounsaturated oils that are thought to provide this protection. The key thing is "one handful"—which is one ounce or one serving. Each serving has 15 grams of fat, so don't subscribe to the idea if one handful is good two should be better. Getting 30 grams of fat from your snack will likely wreck your fat macronutrient range for the day.

Olive oil has long been known to be protective as well but again only in moderate quantities. Flaxseed oil has been shown to decrease cholesterol, and we've seen one to two tablespoons per day help lower cholesterol in some patients and clients. Your personal Rx allows for fat but asks you to keep them unsaturated and on the moderate side for health and more rapid weight loss. Fish, especially salmon and tuna, have naturally occurring omega-3 oils that are very good for the arteries and cerebral function. Concern has been raised about mercury levels in fish, so again moderation is the key to getting proper oils without negative effects.

Saturated fat is always your enemy to a certain degree if you want to have rock-hard abs. People will tell you, "Oh, you just need to exercise more and your stomach will go away." It won't. Fat sits in the layer *under* your skin and *over* your abdominal muscles. You could do 500 crunches a day and if your diet isn't in line, you will do an awful lot of work and still not see the results you desire. I know—I've been there. At times I felt like I lived there.

Now it's time—*past* time to explain which end is up in all of this mayhem.

The Nitty-Gritty

You now know the importance of carbs in fat loss. But dietary fat comes in a close second and actually works hand-in-hand with carbs. As a matter of fact, a physiology professor of Joe's was fond of the saying, "Fat is burned in the flames of carbohydrates." The truth is, you need to have a certain amount of carbohydrates to keep your metabolism normal so you can burn body fat. The metabolism of fat, though, comes with even more misconceptions and misinformation. Fat and carbohydrate intake and their effects on weight loss are very intertwined.

There are two main types of dietary fat: saturated and unsaturated. Saturated fats most commonly come from animal sources. Beef, pork, dairy products, eggs, and poultry all contain saturated fats. Products made with these animal fats—such as butter and cream—are also saturated. Some foods obviously have a great deal more or less fat than others. For example, fish, chicken, and turkey breast have dramatically less fat than beef does.

The problems with saturated fats lie primarily in their structure. They are much larger and more stable than unsaturated fats and, therefore, much harder to break down. Since they don't break down easily, they circulate in the bloodstream longer, create higher blood cholesterol levels, lead to atherosclerosis, and much of it ends up being stored as body fat. There really aren't many positive things to say about saturated fats.

Earlier we mentioned the term "trans-fat." A fat can be classified either as a cis-fat or a trans-fat, depending on its chemical structure. Trans-fats, in general, are those that are solid at room temperature. They are often used in junk food and cheap food

Good Fats/Bad Fats

Unsaturated Fats	Saturated Fats
• Easily used as energy	• Difficult to break down
• Decrease cholesterol	• Increase cholesterol
• Contain essential fatty acids	
• Necessary for many regenerative body processes	
• Necessary to create certain hormones for optimal health, building muscle, and burning body fat	

Figure 3.1

processing. Your cell membranes are made up of fat molecules that create receptor sites (think "ports") for certain chemicals, such as glucose, to be shuttled inside the cells. Trans-fats are rotated and stuck in a "backward" position that doesn't allow this to happen so the cell doesn't function properly. Trans-fats have been linked to cancer as well as heart disease (as with any saturated fat).

Unsaturated fats are found mainly in plant sources such as olive oil, canola oil, flaxseed oil, grapeseed oil, borage oil, some nuts, and in some fish, such as salmon. Molecularly, unsaturated fats are smaller, less stable, and easier to break down. Surprisingly, unsaturated fats have important health benefits and can help you lose body fat! Many unsaturated fats contain specific "essential fatty acids." Each essential fatty acid has unique properties and benefits to the human body. (Notice they're called "essential," a biological term meaning your body can't produce them so you need to supply them.)

Good Fat?

Most people have heard the terms "good fat" and "bad fat." We can assure you that without some unsaturated dietary fat, body fat loss will be slow at first, minimal at best, and ultimately counterproductive.

Some essential fatty acids are the building blocks for certain hormones that control fat loss and storage and the potential for muscle gain and loss. Reread that sentence one more time, please...

Yes, your body produces specific hormones that control how much body fat you can lose or gain and how much muscle you can gain or lose. Your body needs unsaturated fats (essential fatty acids) to create many of these hormones (such as testosterone).

In a matter of weeks, people who consume a no- or low-fat diet start producing less and less of the "good" hormones that promote body fat loss and muscle gain. Conversely, people who consume 20 to 30 percent of their calories from unsaturated fats start producing more of these hormones, often above normal levels. With an increase in your hormonal base, you can actually burn more body fat than normal and build more muscle than normal. Research has

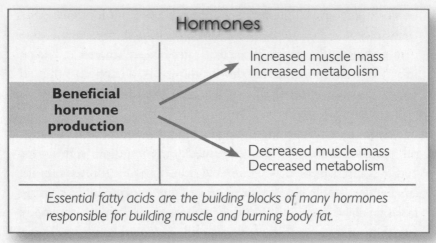

Figure 3.2

demonstrated these incredibly positive blood chemistry changes can lead to decreased cholesterol and increased athletic performance. A little of the *right* dietary fat goes a long way.

We have witnessed dramatic decreases in cholesterol and LDLs (low-density lipoproteins or "bad fat" in the bloodstream) by increasing total dietary fat. We need to qualify this however, with what we see as a very practical aspect of body fat loss and dieting. Most people who are overweight and eating a poor diet often consume too much refined carbohydrates and too much saturated fat. A few hold-overs from the low-fat craze are eating healthy and fall into the category of "need more good fat," but most of us—whether we care to admit it or not—are killing ourselves on both ends. Switching to 20 to 30 percent of calories coming from good fat may cause an overall reduction in body fat. You achieve the best health and best results by eliminating saturated fats and increasing unsaturated fats while keeping carbs in check. You can't leave out carbohydrate control when discussing cholesterol.

Up to 80 percent of your body's cholesterol is produced in your liver as a result of sugar and runaway insulin production. Excess carbohydrates result in a conversion to cholesterol and fat. By recommending a higher intake of unsaturated fats while controlling carbohydrate levels, we have witnessed hypercholesterolemic clients (those whose livers produce a significantly larger amount of cholesterol) lower their cholesterol levels and manage them so well that, under the supervision of their physicians, they've eliminated the use of cholesterol-reducing medications.

One client decreased his blood triglycerides from over 900 to 90 in three months using The Diet Docs' program, along with weight training and cardiovascular exercise. A triglyceride level of 900! His poor heart was pumping pudding, not blood. Diet should be the cornerstone of any cholesterol management program, not an afterthought. If you need medication, take it. Heart disease is serious business. However, cholesterol-lowering medication shouldn't be viewed as a cure or an excuse to not lose weight and exercise.

Saturated Fat Reducing Tips

1. Use nonstick cooking spray to reduce fat or use unsaturated oils to increase "good" fat when cooking.

2. Boil, roast, bake, or steam food in place of frying.

3. Use egg whites in place of whole eggs when baking. Two egg whites equal one whole egg.

4. Use skim milk in place of whole or 2% milk.

5. Choose low- or no-fat yogurts, mayo, and salad dressings.

6. Use spices and fat-free condiments, such as salsa, to spice up food.

7. Use applesauce in place of butter and/or oil in baked goods.

8. Make sure canned tuna, chicken, and other meats are packed in water, not oil.

9. Choose the leanest cuts of meat.

10. Trim fat from meat.

Figure 3.3

Another practical example of the power of correct nutrition is seen in elite athletes whose body composition changes are easily measured and observed. Joe has consulted with and supervised the nutrition of hundreds of bodybuilders, including several world champions preparing for competition. They often need to lose between 15 to 40 pounds of body fat for the contest without losing muscle, and this can certainly be achieved. However, he's also tested the body composition of competitors who were not receiving proper nutritional support, and has been amazed at how much muscle can be lost during dieting—quite a contrast to physiologically sound nutrition.

Burgers and Oils

Consciously switching from saturated to unsaturated fat is a lot easier on paper than in real life. You can switch from a hamburger to a chicken breast or from three whole eggs to six egg whites, but how are you going to get the good fat into your day? The most practical and healthy ways will be to add certain oils to your food. Over time you will naturally start making better food choices and become more creative. For example, if you have a bowl of oatmeal, after it's cooked add one half to a whole tablespoon of flaxseed oil. Do the same thing with brown rice, yogurt, protein shakes, and anything else that can withstand oil without destroying the taste of the food.

If you're making an egg-white omelet, cook it with olive, canola, or grapeseed oil instead of a spray. If salad dressing is where you get some of your fat intake, use an Italian dressing made with olive oil instead of a cream-based dressing with saturated fat. Almonds are a healthy fat source and very practical for a snack.

Differentiating between fats complicates the diet a bit, but "good" fats—essential fatty acids—*must* be integrated into your diet for all of the reasons discussed. They are necessary for your long-term health, for reducing cholesterol, and for creating hormones. Furthermore, a well-placed snack that contains these concentrated healthy fats will sustain energy and decrease hunger longer.

A Little More Detail

A point that must be understood is how dynamic fat is in the body. If you gained 10 pounds last year, you're not retaining the exact same 10 pounds of body fat that was originally stored. Your body is constantly storing triglycerides in adipose (fat) cells and also releasing them as you need more energy between meals. In fact, adipose cells always store fat after meals and then release it when needed. Fat is used for up to 60 percent of the body's energy needs at rest.

A surprising fact to most people is how easily your body stores dietary fat. Dietary fat is the easiest nutrient for your body to store as body fat, which makes sense when you think about it. As the fat from your diet passes by body-fat cells, these cells simply grab the fat and store it. As a matter of fact, when you eat just 3 percent more total calories than your body needs at one time, dietary fat is going to be stored in this manner. However, it takes 25 percent more food than your body needs at one time to start converting excess carbohydrates into body fat. That may sound contradictory as we've made such a big deal of carbohydrates, but don't throw the baby out with the bath water. It's a fact that dietary fat is easier to store as body fat than carbohydrates when calorie intake is more than your body can digest and use at that particular meal. Carbohydrate sources have to be digested, converted into smaller saccharides, dismantled, and then reassembled into fatty acid chains in order to be converted to storable body fat. You need to keep carbs lower and in control to get to accelerated fat loss potential, but you have to keep everything in perspective. Food volume (The Diet Docs' Rx) is step one, power spacing is step two, carb quality and quantity is step three, and then fat closely follows in importance.

If you're tracking this data carefully, you'll see why we said that overall calorie intake is still always the first step. Total calorie consumption is taken care of by eating within the boundaries of your personal macronutrient range as indicated on the all-important chart in chapter 5. If you're taking in a moderate amount of fat, even unsaturated fats, a great deal of it can end up stored as fat *if* carbs and/or overall calories are too high (remember the 3 percent rule from the last paragraph). However, if your overall calorie intake is lower than your metabolic rate requires, you'll end up using that dietary fat as well as stored fat between meals.

You might ask, if so much of dietary fat ends up being stored as body fat, why not eliminate it completely? Essential fatty acids play a role in hormone production as well as cellular repair, immune function, and many other life processes. If you are deficient in essential fatty acids, health consequences cumulatively add physical stress to your body. Another key reason is the focus on keeping blood sugar moderated. Fat takes longer to digest and slows the digestion and assimilation of carbohydrates, so insulin spiking is less of a problem. This type of fat intake has merit, but only if the percentages are representative of an overall calorie intake that's low enough to cause a caloric deficit.

As already discussed in detail, the relationship between fats and carbohydrates is very important. If fat intake, for example, is 25 percent of the total calories instead of 15 percent, a little lower carbohydrate intake will be necessary to accommodate the additional dietary fat. However, lowering the carbohydrates may then make the practicality of healthy food intake difficult and energy levels may drop. Thus, a slightly lower fat intake that allows for more carbohydrates may be necessary. Some flexibility between carbohydrates and fat is allowed in the Diet Docs' Rx, and you should feel comfortable trying different combinations as long as you stay within both ranges.

A discussion of fat intake and dietary theory wouldn't be complete without commenting on the ketogenic (low-carb) camp. What do we do with the "experts" that promise us a lean, muscular physique if we eat unlimited amounts of fat and protein but eschew carbs?

Since excess carbs are easily converted to body fat and lead to insulin-induced lethargy, higher risk of diabetes and heart disease, and many other health perils, it's good to control carbs and their

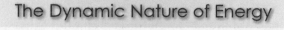

The Dynamic Nature of Energy

- Blood sugar too low
- Glucagon released
- Glycogen harvested
- Fat released

Body Fat Cell

- Blood sugar too high
- Insulin released
- Glycogen stored
- Fat stored

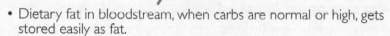

- Dietary fat in bloodstream, when carbs are normal or high, gets stored easily as fat.
- Dietary fat in bloodstream, when carbs are low, gets converted and used as glucose in place of stored body fat.

Figure 3.4

quality. It's also imperative to make sure that your carb intake is low enough to *not* supply all the energy requirements of your body.

A high-carb diet in which protein and fat intake is low doesn't allow for much fat loss because the body will have little reason to access a secondary energy source, such as body fat.

If you take the opposite extreme and eliminate most carbohydrates from the body, stored fat will be released at a very rapid rate. Though seemingly used successfully by many bodybuilders, this type of dieting has problems. First, adipose cells release fat to be used as energy in the form of glycerol and fatty acids. Body cells intake the glycerol and fatty acids to metabolize them into energy through what's called "Kreb's cycle," but glucose fragments *must* be present. (Hmm…looks like Joe's physiology professor was right, fat is burned in the flames of carbohydrates.)

Glucose fragments (carbs) must be present to burn body fat for energy through the very efficient Kreb's cycle within every cell. But Kreb's cycle isn't the only way. If glucose isn't available, fatty acids can combine with each other to form "ketone" bodies that can also be used by most cells for energy conversion. This is the goal of low-carb diets. The rate of body fat usage for energy can be great using this method of diet, but what are the negatives?

Ketogenic (low-carb) dieting may be effective only if fat intake isn't excessive. Remember, adipose cells are just waiting to suck in new fat to store after meals. One of the two greatest problems of low-carb dieting is that if carbs are too low for too long, you'll lose muscle no matter how much protein you eat.

Second, the brain and nervous system prefer glucose, not ketone bodies, for energy. Low energy and inefficient nervous system activity make workouts low-key, weak, and less effective. And you'll experience fatigue in daily life.

So if you enjoy feeling lousy, having no energy, craving carbohydrates intensely, and being prone to bingeing, low-carb dieting is for you. Ketogenic dieting certainly allows you to burn more fat initially because of the immense carb deficit, but increasing fat intake too much can cause a great deal of fat storage. Two steps forward, two steps back. The few who have successfully employed this type of dieting leave me wondering how much easier it would have been had they used better dieting principles in the first place.

What's the take-home message about fat? If you're in a maintaining stage of nondieting, you can successfully eat 30 percent or more of your calories from fat sources without a problem—though I would choose approximately 20 percent of the total so that more protein and/or carbs can be consumed. The key is "isocaloric," eating the same amount of total calories that your body uses for energy so that you won't store new body fat.

Carbohydrate control and planning are just as important as dietary fat. The two go hand-in-hand.

Many people who obsess about carbs alone end up snacking on too many nuts, extra peanut butter, and other high-fat, low-carb foods, and increase direct fat storage from the increased fat intake. When taking in a limited amount of fat, be sure to make the most of what you get and supplement with essential fatty acids. Don't lose

Average Joe Physiology

Avoid Fat Altogether?

The question of which is worse—excess dietary fat or excess carbohydrates in relation to cardiovascular disease—is still largely misunderstood. Even if you're only 20 years old, this is an important concept to understand completely. Coronary artery blockage often invokes the imagery of some fatty deposits that can be scoured away with proper eating and exercise. The truth is that the atherosclerotic fat that collects on the artery walls starts a process that isn't entirely reversible. The plaque that forms creates an inflammatory condition by which collagen also collects, creating a fibrous lesion. Even as plaque and cholesterol are reduced through diet and exercise, some narrowing of the vessels remains permanent. The answer is to be responsible and heart-healthy early in life and keep it up.

The average American diet includes 40 percent of calories from fat. Though 20 to 30 percent is more appropriate, that still leaves a large amount of calories that you can choose from unsaturated, natural sources or from saturated and trans-fatty acids. Obviously the latter will perpetuate the process of heart disease, but many choose another avenue of proactive dieting. Some are swayed to decrease overall fat consumption to as low as possible and eat more carbohydrates to replace those calories. Studies show that type of dieting can lower LDL-cholesterol levels, but it also tends to lower "good" HDL-cholesterol levels and can increase triglyceride levels. When replacing carbohydrates with monounsaturated natural oils, studies show a decrease in triglycerides and an increase in HDLs. Polyunsaturated oils did decrease LDLs but didn't have much of an effect on HDLs or triglycerides. For heart health, the best combination is to keep carbohydrates low enough so that saturated fats can be replaced by some monounsaturated fats. (Olive oil and almonds are two of the richest sources of monounsaturated fats.)

sight of the big picture: Dietary fat intake control is a critical part of your success, but it has to be just one piece of a comprehensive plan to work.

One last word about fats: Have a steak once in a while (unless you're a vegetarian…in which case, have a tofu steak….or whatever your favorite meal is). A small percentage of saturated fat isn't going to throw you into cardiac arrest, and if your cholesterol is too low, you can suffer from low energy, low hormonal levels, and even depression. This is admittedly rare, but it does happen, especially with those who are very disciplined and deep into a weight-loss cycle.

Key Points

1. Saturated fats are found primarily in animal sources.

2. Saturated fats lead to heart disease and body fat.

3. Unsaturated fats contain essential fatty acids that are necessary for many body processes.

4. Unsaturated fats in the right amounts are necessary to lose the maximal amount of body fat and to build muscle.

The Diet Docs in Action...

Randy and Debbie's Stories

Randy

Wow! Thank you, thank you, thank you, Diet Docs! Talk about an easy program to follow for an old German. At 55, I didn't think I would ever be able to change my eating habits. I like food too much, and I enjoy preparing it as well. But over the years the pounds added up, and in 2002 my weight peaked at 285 pounds on my 5'11" frame. I dropped about 50 pounds over the next year on a diabetic diet, having been diagnosed with Type II Diabetes that year by Dr. Uloth. But old habits die hard, and I was soon back up to 260 pounds. More health problems developed, along with herniated discs that required steroid injections.

Dr. Uloth kept after me to go see Dr. Joe, but this stubborn idiot kept thinking, *Nah, I can do it myself.* But, you know, it takes a good coach to lead you to success in anything in life that is worth doing well. As a former athlete, I remembered the importance of practice and being focused on a certain goal, as well as working together as a team. With Dr. Joe, Dr. Uloth, my wife, and me on this team, I knew success was sure to come—and it has.

My wife and I decided to change our lifelong eating habits to improve our health. We wanted to see our grandchildren grow up and marry and be able to share with them what we were learning. So after just three months on The Diet Docs' program, I have lost 48 pounds and haven't started an exercise program of any kind as of yet. My glycated hemoglobin has dropped from 6.5 in September to 5.9. I have lost four inches off my waist and dropped one complete shirt size. My blood pressure is back to a more manageable level, and my back pain has started to ease. We'll be beginning our exercise training soon and look forward to the added success that I know will come.

I sincerely hope that men who read this book will give up trying to be "real men" and just for once in their lives listen to the coach! And believe me, Dr. Joe is a great coach.

Debbie

Randy and I have enough health problems between us that our medical records read like a medical school textbook. We love to eat, cook, and entertain. In fact, most of our social activities seem centered around food.

continued →

A natural result of this lifestyle, accompanied with no exercise, is that we both became obese. Our family physician, Dr. Scott Uloth, encouraged us for years to contact Dr. Joe and to read their book.

In 2007 our granddaughter, Ava, was born. We were excited, but facing our own serious health problems. Our desire to watch her grow up was the motivation to do what we needed to do all along.

We started the program on September 30, 2007. By March 1, 2008, only 5 months into it, I have lost 70 pounds and Randy, 48 pounds. We have more energy and feel better than we have in years, and we have not been hungry. The food diaries, which I detested at first, have been the most valuable tool in deciding what to eat when and making healthy food choices when eating out.

It feels good when we hear our friends tell us we look great. More importantly, we both can say we feel great!

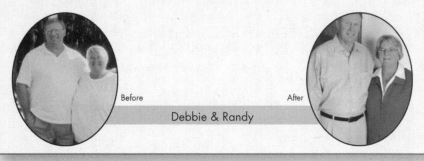

Before   After

Debbie & Randy

CHAPTER 4

Power to the Proteins

Just as most saturated fats come from animal sources, so does most protein. We need protein, but we don't want saturated fat. "Houston, we have a problem." But thankfully, fish, chicken and turkey breasts, egg whites, and even soy-based meat substitutes are alternatives to foods high in saturated fat, such as beef, pork, dairy products, and whole eggs. These healthier foods are now commonly found in most restaurants, making them easier to obtain on the go.

Another convenient protein choice comes in the form of protein powders, shakes, and bars. The reason professional athletes endorse supplement companies (besides getting paid) is that they use their products.

Getting supplemental protein in the form of a great tasting shake or bar, especially in on-the-run situations, is easy. We couldn't eat properly and still see a high volume of patients and clients without an occasional bar or shake to supplement our whole-food meals. Getting some of your protein from these sources will also help you avoid feeling like you're growing a beak from eating so much poultry.

Why Protein?

Most bodybuilders would correctly tell you that you need protein to build muscle. They would probably also tell you, incorrectly, that you need two to three times what you really require. If you asked a vegetarian about protein, you might learn how to make a dozen eggs last for a year. Your body has the ability to survive either extreme, but you will pay the price for each. You can survive without much protein at all, but you will strip the muscle right off your bones and impair your ability to build the healthiest cells.

Consume too much protein, as advocated by some muscle magazines (owned by protein supplement companies), and you may spend a lifetime in a state of acidosis, creating a host of degenerative diseases. Some experts warn you could also end up on the kidney transplant waiting list. How much protein is best?

The amount of protein we advocate is designed to abundantly meet the body's requirements without the risk of undesirable effects. Protein is very important in creating new cells—red blood cells, skin cells, liver cells, etc.—as well as fueling the maintenance and metabolic activities of every system in your body. If protein intake is too low, your entire body eventually suffers, even your immune system.

At first you can withstand protein depletion because you have so much stored. Protein is broken down into amino acids, which are used in just about every chemical reaction that takes place within your body. Amino acids are made up of nitrogen compounds that circulate in your bloodstream and are stored in a few places, mostly as skeletal muscle and some in the liver. You can live a long time without protein, and even longer with insufficient amounts of protein. Your body will simply break down your muscle tissue to provide what it needs. It's a great survival mechanism, but you don't want to knowingly lose any muscle.

Our protein estimates in the Diet Docs' Rx are for active people (see chapter 5). If you aren't performing rigorous exercise at least three to four times per week, choose the lower end of suggested protein ranges shown on the chart. If you train extremely hard or perform several sessions of cardiovascular work per week, you may need to go slightly above the suggested amount.

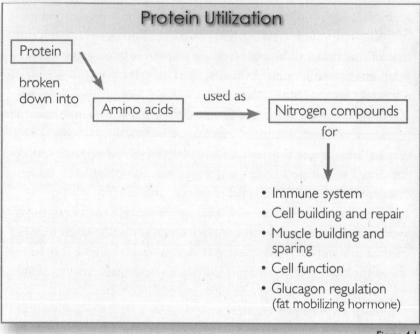

Protein Utilization

Protein

broken
down into → Amino acids

used as →

Nitrogen compounds

for ↓

• Immune system
• Cell building and repair
• Muscle building and sparing
• Cell function
• Glucagon regulation (fat mobilizing hormone)

Figure 4.1

Variety Is the Spice of Life

Every protein has a specific amino acid profile. This means each protein source may be higher or lower in certain amino acids than other protein sources. There are many rating scales that attempt to build a hierarchy among protein sources by assigning values and deeming them "high-" or "low-quality" protein sources. There is merit to these types of ratings. However, even the highest-rated protein source is low in certain amino acids.

If you're a vegetarian, you may have also heard that you have to combine certain foods to "make a complete protein." You're covered on this principle on two different fronts. First, digestion, absorption, and circulation keep the amino acids that you consume available for hours, and they can be augmented with other amino acids in previous or later meals. The liver also stores a small reserve of amino acids that it uses when necessary.

While we're on the subject of protein and vegetarianism, we want to make sure you understand you can succeed on our program without animal protein. We still recommend getting at least the minimal suggested protein intake in your Diet Docs' Rx for all the reasons discussed so far. Think about it: If you avoid protein as a vegetarian, most of your food will come from carbohydrates, causing the same physiological and behavioral challenges to health and weight loss. We have had many vegetarian clients lose weight, drop their cholesterol, and regain surprising energy by trimming starch and adding a couple of protein shakes or other protein source daily.

The bottom line is to enjoy a variety of protein sources throughout your day so you take in a variety of amino acids. Keep in mind that saturated fats should be kept to a minimum so your diet leaves room for high-quality unsaturated fats and essential fatty acids.

Back to Hormones

Just as carbohydrates can affect your body in a positive or negative way through the modulation of the hormone insulin, protein creates a similar effect through the hormone glucagon. In simple terms, insulin is released when you eat carbs; glucagon is released when you eat protein. Just as insulin is a storage hormone, glucagon is a retrieval, or mobilizing, hormone. It promotes glucose to be used as energy. When glucose isn't present in large enough quantities (because you've been so good at limiting your carbs and sticking to your daily totals!), glucagon helps mobilize body fat to be burned as energy. That's why it's important to break your daily macronutrient totals up so you have protein in most meals.

Average Joe Physiology

Why Protein Helps

High-protein, low-carb diets have cycled into the diet fad rotation about every 20 years since the 1950s. Though we can all agree that carbohydrates are a critical—maybe the most important—variable in dieting, it can be taken to an unhealthy and even dangerous level. Many of these diets allow unlimited amounts of protein as long as carbs stay ultra-low. Naysayers claim that too high of a protein intake can be stressful to the kidneys, but however logical, very little evidence exists to support kidney damage. Yet there are other reasons to avoid this extreme approach.

First, studies show a very high incidence of weight regain, often with decreased lean body mass. Eliminating carbohydrates will reduce blood levels of insulin—a very good thing—but to such a low level that your body becomes insulin sensitive. A significant hormone, adipsin, works inside the body fat cell to help regulate how much blood glucose will get pulled into the cell to be stored as fat. Its activation is modulated by insulin. Since ketogenic metabolism is less efficient than glucose metabolism, the body becomes more sensitive to glucose as it desperately wants to use it for energy. When in this hypersensitive state, the hormone adipsin has been measured to be many times more effective at storing glucose as body fat. This is the basis of the "starvation mode" cliché often used as an excuse for not losing weight. The truth is, you have to be consuming virtually no carbohydrates for approximately eight weeks to have an appreciable change, but if you remain on a very low carb diet, increased adipsin sensitivity will happen. The body literally becomes a fat-storing machine. The process will reverse itself as carbohydrate intake increases, but in the meantime, much body fat may be regained.

The second most important reason to avoid low-carb diets is the negative effect they have on mood and brain function. The brain cannot use free fatty acids for energy, has very little amounts of glycogen stored, and consumes a whopping 20 percent of the body's total energy at rest. It can use ketone bodies as energy in a fasting state, but mental function is greatly compromised. Eating moderate carbs is a prescription for success as well as for a sharp noodle!

Think of insulin and glucagon as representing two opposite metabolic stimuli. Insulin is present, active, and dominant if carbohydrate intake is too high. Your body is in storage mode. Glucagon is present, active, and dominant when carbohydrate intake is lower and protein intake is higher, thus promoting fat mobilization. Glucagon is one of several hormones that can "unlock" body fat cells and is the most powerful that is nutrition dependent. Others are more exercise dependent. When you combine the most effective nutrition and exercise to maximize these hormones, you truly are working with your body for the fastest progress.

Protein also has the greatest "thermic potential" among macronutrients. This means that when you eat protein, your metabolism rises because protein digestion requires more energy. Protein is very important for health and body composition, but in most cases it is deficient in the American diet. This, along with hormonal considerations such as glucagon, is the reason many new studies are showing that diets higher in protein and lower (notice we say "lower" and not "low") in carbs can cause twice as much body fat loss—even with the same amount of calories!

If you're "starving" and just have to have a little more food on a particular day than your macronutrient range allows, it's better to eat a little more protein than to end up bingeing. But if you do this too often you'll find overall calories too high and insulin will be a factor in keeping you from losing as much weight.

You must have lean protein...with the emphasis on "lean." Eating protein indiscriminately can cause problems. Don't get too much of a good thing. If you eat an excessive amount of protein—calories are calories—insulin can be stimulated, so be careful. But most people don't take in sufficient protein. Adults need about 50 to 70 grams a day for body function, and many of us, especially women, may only get 30 to 40 grams a day. This is part of the reason why in our mid-thirties we start to lose about half a pound of lean muscle a year. (The other part is lack of exercise.) You need lean protein combined with exercise to keep your muscles strong.

Key Points

1. Protein is found in animal meats and in small amounts in certain plants, including beans.

2. Supplemental protein can be found in many types of protein shakes and bars.

3. Protein is necessary for many vital processes in the body, including muscle growth.

4. Protein sources have different amino acid profiles, making it advantageous to vary your protein choices.

5. Eating protein raises your metabolism, and through the actions of the hormone glucagon, assists you in losing body fat faster.

CHAPTER 5

The Diet Docs' Rx

Okay, now you know what the three macronutrients are—carbohydrates, fats, and proteins. The next step—and the key to losing weight effectively—is learning how to daily apportion the macronutrients in such a way as to instruct your body to start drawing on its stored fat for energy instead of turning your food into *more* stored fat.

To know how to choose the right amount of macronutrients, you must determine the right amount of food necessary to reach your goal. To that end, we've developed a chart based on gender and height to make this most important step very easy. This all-important chart (Figure 5.1, p.71) is your roadmap to successful weight loss. Please make sure you understand how to use it. It is the centerpiece of the Diet Docs' plan.

As you tailor your meals to correspond to the chart, *you will lose weight*. And it won't be long before you will learn the amounts of each macronutrient your body needs to maintain your desired weight.

This chart ensures enough food to avoid any deficiencies in the three macronutrients and is geared toward a one-to-two pound weight loss per week. A great deal of experience and human trial has been poured into this chart to make it a simple yet potent weapon in your battle for permanent weight control. For some readers it may seem too easy to just plug yourself into a chart and follow the numbers, but therein lies the challenge. You will need discipline to follow the chart.

Most people won't have a clear concept regarding the numbers on the chart. That is, most can't at first glance correlate how much food is required to eat 100 grams of protein or even what foods contain protein. But fear not! Within six weeks you will be well on the way to knowing this, to becoming your own nutritionist.

Thousands of clients have found this plan provides the most attainable and sustainable results they've ever experienced. And a huge plus is the flexibility you have in food selection, along with the guidance given in your personal macronutrient range profile. Again, *this Diet Docs' Rx chart is the cornerstone of the program.*

Figure 5.2 is where you will enter the appropriate amounts for your personal Rx. We advise making a photocopy of Figure 5.2 and keeping it with you until you have developed the habit of staying within your allowable range.

Now you have one of our most powerful tools, and we didn't make you wait 20 chapters to find it! Those of you who wanted something simple, here it is: Eat within the levels appropriate for your gender and height as indicated on the chart and you'll lose weight. Thank you and good night.

We both understand, however, that healthy eating and losing weight is more than just hitting a gram or calorie total. Knowing what to eat, structuring your day nutritionally, planning meals, and learning about the individuality of your body is what will pay dividends long after you put this book aside.

Everything from this point on originates from this one simple step of consuming the right amounts of the three macronutrients. I'll provide a great deal of information that will make this one step even easier, yet it will ultimately be your responsibility to stay within the levels on this chart.

The Diet Docs' Rx (Personal Macronutrient Range)		
	Men	Women
Height	(Grams per day)	
Under 5'		
Protein	100–120	60–80
Carbohydrates	120–150	80–110
Fat	35–40	20–25
(Calories)	(1,195–1,440)	(740–985)
5'– 5'4"		
Protein	110 130	70–90
Carbohydrates	130–160	90–120
Fat	40–45	25–30
(Calories)	(1,320–1,565)	(865–1,110)
5'5"– 5'8"		
Protein	120–140	80–100
Carbohydrates	140–170	100–130
Fat	45–50	30–35
(Calories)	(1,445–1,690)	(990–1,235)
5'9"– 6'		
Protein	130–150	90–110
Carbohydrates	150–180	110–140
Fat	50–55	35–40
(Calories)	(1,570–1,815)	(1,115–1,360)
6'1"– 6'4"		
Protein	140–160	100–120
Carbohydrates	160–190	120–150
Fat	55–60	40–45
(Calories)	(1,695–1,940)	(1,240–1,485)

Figure 5.1

My Personal Rx
(grams/day)

Protein _____

Carbs _____

Fat _____

- Document everything.
- Only one "splurge" meal per week (not a day or a weekend or…).
- Eat five to six times per day (three meals and two to three snacks).
- Eat even if you don't feel hungry initially to prevent bingeing ("stay ahead of hunger").
- Weigh/measure your food initially (make sure an ounce is an ounce, a cup is a cup).
- Read labels carefully and watch portion size.
- Exercise five to six times per week and try to strength train at least two of those days.
- Keep constantly armed with good foods.

Figure 5.2

Doing so won't require weird foods (like pomegranates or grilled alligator) or crazy behaviors (like sit-ups hanging from your garage rafters or pushing a cart through snowy Russian mountains as seen in *Rocky IV*). You'll just need *discipline*. There are two very different definitions for the word "discipline." The first is punishment. As soon as you read the word "discipline" related to weight loss, it sounds like punishment. However, the second definition is *your* definition for this program: to train or develop by instruction; to impose order upon; orderly or prescribed conduct or pattern of behavior.

That doesn't sound too hard, does it?

We want to train you in new habits that maximize your effort and health. To do so takes order. You need to learn a new pattern of behavior. We'll give you the prescription, and with the right motivation, we know you'll happily follow it with the promise of permanent weight loss and a healthier body.

We've established that everyone is different metabolically. Our chart, which was created for people with moderate activity levels, may not be a perfect fit for a few readers. For most, the goal of losing as much as five to seven pounds the first week due to water loss and one to two pounds each week thereafter is realistic.

If you don't obtain the desired results despite following your allowable food totals perfectly, eating the best food selections as described, and using the methods in this book, you may need to make an adjustment (Flexibility alert!).

First, if you are not losing weight fast enough (one to two pounds per week), make sure you're eating at the low end of your macronutrient range. If you're losing too rapidly, make sure you're eating at the high end. If you're *still* losing too fast, add 25 grams of carbohydrates to your daily totals for a week and reassess your results. Keep adding until you are losing at the desired rate. If you're still losing too slowly even at the low end of your suggested chart totals, drop your daily intake of carbs by 10 grams daily for a week and reassess. If necessary, repeat this until you're losing weight at the appropriate rate.

The importance of the macronutrient ranges *(The Diet Docs' Rx)* is its simplicity that allows you to get a running start on losing weight. However, we want you to become your own nutritionist and ask, "Is this something that I really want to put in my body?" when faced with choices. No longer is it adequate for a physician to tell us that we "need to lose a few pounds." This program gives you an actual plan to accomplish that goal.

How It Works

Not long ago a 44-year-old man came to Joe with a goal of getting leaner and possibly gaining some muscle. He was an active man who was already working out and running almost daily, and had been for most of his adult life. Despite his good health and his exercise habits, he'd gained and lost 20 pounds several times. He wanted to lose weight again, but this time he wanted the weight loss to be permanent.

"What can you do to help me?" he asked. He suggested Joe could hypnotize him and plant subconscious links between snack cakes and rat poison. However, the greatest pathway to success is to help people get their metabolism in order and then teach them how to maintain it.

There is an intertwining of the physiological and psychological aspects of weight loss that can't be separated. Many failed dieters feel tremendous guilt about their perceived lack of discipline, but their real problem may simply be they don't understand how their individual metabolism works and what they can do to positively affect it.

We can't tell you how many times we've heard, "I have control over every aspect of my life except my weight. Why?" The physical and mental aspects of weight control affect each other in a very dynamic way. As you'll learn in the rest of this chapter, the first week of changing your nutritional habits brings about significant changes in your body internally; literally creating stability that makes it easier than you think to not only lose weight, but to do it without suffering. "Attainable and sustainable" is the phrase you can use to describe *The Diet Docs' Rx*.

In his first 8 weeks on our plan, Joe's new client lost 20 pounds of body fat and gained 5 pounds of lean muscle mass. How can a man who already exercises regularly, works out with weights at least four days per week, and runs in road races have such dramatic results just by changing his nutrition?

The answer is metabolism. This man actually complained of having to eat so much food on our plan (his program), yet after those first eight weeks he had to *further* increase his food so he wouldn't lose weight too quickly. During this time he often remarked about his new, higher level of energy. A very disciplined, in-control person, he went so far as to say, "Coming to you literally changed my life."

Is that comment typical of dieters you know? Not likely. Study after study has shown most dieters eventually regain even more weight than they lost on any given plan. We are here to break that mold! We're going to set you up for permanent results, not just a temporary fix.

How many times have you heard people say they have a fast or slow metabolism? Thin people often say, "I have a fast metabolism," and those who are overweight often say, "I have a slow metabolism." We're quick to blame or credit our body size based on a word most of us don't really understand.

Basal metabolic rate (see Figure 5.3) is how much your body burns calories over a specific amount of time. It's true that there's some variability in metabolism. We have met a few people who had a legitimately slow metabolism due to a thyroid imbalance, metabolic condition, and medical ailments that would compromise weight loss. In other words, your metabolism may be slightly lower than someone else's, but it's probably *not* the reason you're overweight.

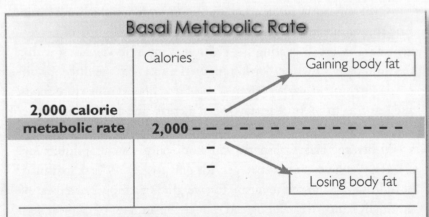

Eating fewer calories than the body needs is the first step to losing weight. However, if done improperly the body will decrease calorie burning, making it easier to gain body fat. Permanent, positive changes in metabolism occur through the combined results of eating nutrients in the right amounts in a structured meal plan.

Figure 5.3

More likely, the cause of your weight struggle goes beyond metabolism; though for a small percentage of people, genetics do play a major role in making it easier to gain or lose weight. Hormone levels that were not measurable for a long time are now being found to be major players in weight loss and gain. These hormones directly control metabolism, fat storage, and even hunger levels. The number of fat cells can even vary significantly between people, making it harder for some to lose weight. But the sad truth for most of us is that we're overweight due to our eating habits. For those few who truly are challenged at the gene-level, there is great research being done on morbid (extreme) obesity that may eventually produce helpful breakthroughs.

Don't misunderstand. While we're downplaying the role of metabolism as an excuse for failing to lose weight, we heartily agree that it does play a great role with long-term impact in the big picture of weight management. And what you eat *does* affect your metabolism. Within weeks, you can raise or lower your body's ability to burn calories, sometimes significantly.

Over time, this change can add up to large weight loss or gain. And this bodily function of metabolism is the foundation of permanent weight loss. By eating the right amount of food, eating within the right daily structure, consuming better ratios of the three macronutrients (protein, carbohydrates, and fat), choosing the right foods, and learning to be consistent, you can increase the amount of calories your body burns per day.

When you diet improperly, your body can't work at optimum levels. The dieter who has lost 30 pounds only to gain 40 back may insist he didn't gorge himself to regain the weight but simply started eating "normally." Incorrect dieting can reduce the amount of calories your body burns, making it much easier to gain weight even though you're still trying to lose. Pay close attention to the details in this chapter as we explore how your body works with healthy eating and diet.

Average Joe Physiology

The Straight Scoop on Metabolism

Numerous studies show how quickly our bodies can be affected by changes in diet. The dreaded "slow metabolism" isn't to be blamed by most of us. The super-sized lunches, chips, snacks, double helpings at dinner, and the worn track from the couch to the kitchen are the real culprits. But when we choose to embark on a weight-loss plan, we can do some short-term damage to our metabolism by incorrect eating.

A study showed that after 24 days of low-calorie dieting (450 calories—that's low!) the metabolism can be decreased by 15 percent. Several studies have reported decreases in resting metabolic rate up to 20 to 30 percent. Dropping your metabolism that fast means you're likely to regain more weight back when you start "eating normally" until your metabolism catches back up, which it will do. In extreme cases, such as anorexia, metabolic rates have been slashed by 45 percent.

You may not be aware that just as eating too little decreases your metabolic rate, overeating increases it. This is where we lose the "I'm fat because of a slow metabolism" excuse. One study showed that when subjects who required 3,100 calories to maintain their weight gained 20 percent or more of their initial weight, they had to eat 5,100 calories to maintain that extra weight due to a heightened metabolism. (That gives credence to some who say, "I don't eat enough, that's why I can't lose weight.") Metabolism is very sensitive and needs to sometimes be "rebuilt," but changes have to be made incrementally.

The importance of small changes can be shown clearly by contrasting the negative results of yo-yo dieting. Going on and off diets repeatedly makes it more difficult to lose weight. Remember, the negative effects are short-term, and your metabolism can be corrected, but the damage (weight regain) can be done so fast that you regain more weight than you lost. One study took subjects through two cycles of weight loss and weight regain. The rate of loss was only half during the second cycle compared to the first and the rate of regain was increased by 300 percent! That means when you diet and then binge and then diet again, you are only 50 percent as effective metabolically than the first round, and when your metabolism

continued ⟶

is suppressed from the dieting, you regain weight back three times faster than if you hadn't dieted at all. (That's how sensitive your metabolism is and why you need to have a knowledge base to guide you to successful and permanent weight loss.)

Scott learned this fact the hard way over the holidays when we first worked together. Already doing well with his weight loss, he thought, *Hey, I'm exercising. I'm doing well. I can eat all this sugar and fat and just burn it off.* One dessert led to another, party after party, and 17 pounds later reality set in. It took months to re-lose that weight, and he learned that he couldn't outsmart his metabolism!

Eating the Right Amount

As we progress, you'll clearly see how the amount, type, and pattern of food consumption can literally accelerate your metabolism to full throttle. The first and most important step is to correctly estimate your metabolic rate so you can eat the right amount of food that will allow you to reach your weight-loss goal. Knowing how much energy your body requires allows you to adjust your eating to begin the weight-loss process.

You might logically assume that eating 5 calories less than your body requires burns 5 extra calories stored as body fat or that if you consume 500 calories less, your body makes up the difference by burning 500 calories of stored fat. But actually the process is more complex than this. There's far more to permanent weight loss than reducing calories. For instance, the body can burn calories by catabolizing (breaking down) other tissues such as muscle. Even if your goals don't include gaining muscle, the last thing you want to do is lose lean body mass through catabolization. Retaining muscle is too important for long-term metabolic function, strength, energy, and even in preventing osteoporosis. Other "intermediate" sources of energy such as blood sugar and stored carbohydrates (glycogen) in the liver and muscle may be used as well. *The goal is to maximize fat loss while sparing muscle.* There's a fine line between losing the most body fat as fast as possible and doing it in such a way so as to not lower your metabolism.

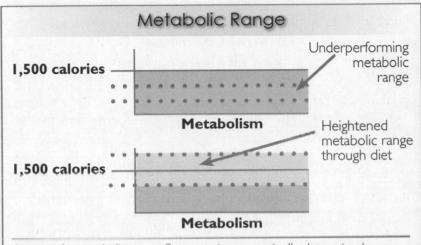

A person's metabolism can fluctuate in a genetically determined range. It doesn't stay the same but can be influenced by diet and exercise. When dieting, the right volume and range of proteins, carbohydrates, and fat can keep it as high as possible.

Figure 5.4

What to Expect the First Week

As you decrease your carbs and are creating the habit to get adequate protein in your diet, you may have a few days of feeling run down. There shouldn't be an overwhelming number of those days. Typically they pass in less than a week. This is another benefit of a nutrition plan based on health instead of a whacky diet. You will not be asked to run like a sports car into a brick wall by cutting your usual 300 carbs a day to 25 overnight. Ask any of your Atkinsian friends (is that like Dickensian? "Please, sir, can I have some more butter on my steak?") how well their brain functioned on 25 carbs a day or how long they were able to sustain it. When you follow The Diet Docs' Rx and consume a reasonable amount of carbs with protein, you'll have a good level of energy and your hunger will be very manageable. If you ever experience a tiny hunger pang at the end of the evening it may signal that you will have a good morning on the scale, so don't grab a snack and go to bed overly full and then watch those little red numbers go up in the morning. Furthermore, hunger will truly fade as your body transitions to faster levels of body fat loss.

For my soda-guzzling friends: You folks have to get off the sauce! Many of us cite the inevitable "caffeine headache" as to why we don't stop our habit. There are 40 to 45 carbs in a 12-ounce can and a mind-numbing 75 grams in a 20-ounce bottle, which is 30 to 50 percent of what your daily carb intake should be. A 44-ounce convenience-store fountain drink has enough sugar to power a small country! If you're truly serious about losing weight, you must kick the soda habit. You really won't be able to afford even one can a day on our nutritionally balanced program. That huge sugar load will send your insulin levels through the roof and will lead to fat storage. One study shows that merely one can a day of regular pop can cause you to gain 15 pounds over the course of a year. Even more serious is the impact on your pancreas and insulin receptor sites. The constant sugar loading may seem like a harmless habit, but you're laying the groundwork for diabetes. So don't "Do the Dew"!

Scott found that when he ate enough protein during the day, he never got a caffeine headache. He didn't like coffee or tea so he never substituted with those. We believe some of the headaches people experience are actually hypoglycemia, and when their blood sugar is better balanced, they don't have as severe a problem with withdrawal headaches. Scott once asked my friends who had been engineers at a soda manufacturing company if they put something addictive in their product, and they said, "Yeah, sugar and caffeine." "No way, my learned friends," he said. "There must be some kind of secret addictive ingredient, a chemical X, that keeps you hooked." "Yeah," they said, "sugar and caffeine." Work on getting rid of soda and other sugary drinks. Watch out for juice drinks or other products that masquerade as "healthy" yet have as much or more carbs than soda. Water is the healthiest drink you can put in your body. There is indeed a reason that your body and this planet are made up of so much of it—it's good for you!

As mentioned earlier, your body has many sources of energy to draw from. As you lower your calorie intake below what's necessary (your basal metabolic rate), the caloric deficit must be made up from somewhere. Though we would all like it to be body fat that's used

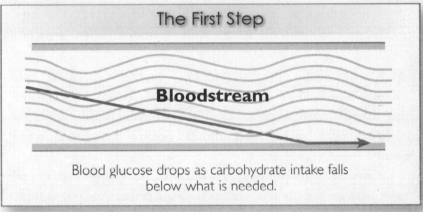

The First Step

Bloodstream

Blood glucose drops as carbohydrate intake falls below what is needed.

Figure 5.5

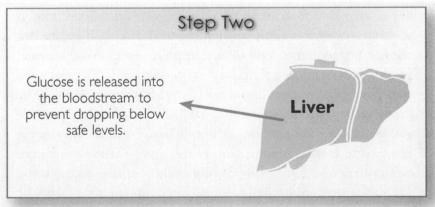

Step Two

Glucose is released into the bloodstream to prevent dropping below safe levels.

Liver

Figure 5.6

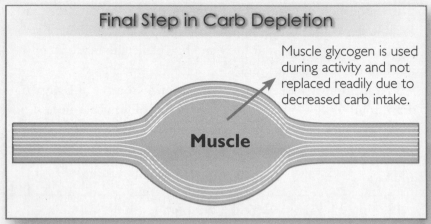

Figure 5.7

up, there is actually a percentage of energy taken from almost every available source. The most readily available source is blood sugar and then liver glycogen (stored sugar). These are dynamic, easy-to-access energy supplies that are tapped into immediately by your body when needed.

Muscle glycogen is a large area of stored energy; however, its primary purpose is for muscle contraction and is therefore not as easily retrieved for maintenance caloric needs. Between meals, body fat is released from body-fat cells, but only as much as needed.

This information is monumental to your understanding, so follow closely. Your food intake is now precise and consistent so that you will get precise and consistent results. The total amount of calories is moderately *lower* than your body needs on a daily basis so that it now requires a secondary source of calories. The first place your body goes to access those calories is blood sugar, followed by liver glycogen, and then by a moderate amount of available muscle glycogen (especially if you work out). The Diet Docs' Rx chart is designed to make a large portion of the caloric deficit come from carbohydrates so that as long as your body continues to use blood sugar and glycogen, you will eventually (within two to four days) be as carb-depleted as your brain will safely allow. This can end up as

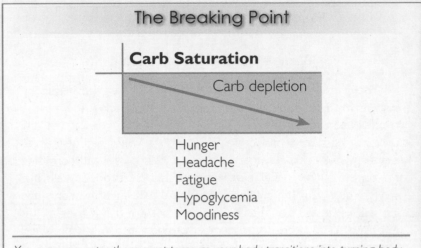

The Breaking Point

Carb Saturation

Carb depletion

Hunger
Headache
Fatigue
Hypoglycemia
Moodiness

You may encounter these symptoms as your body transitions into turning body fat into glucose, but they will be brief because the carb count provided in the Diet Docs' Rx is moderate, not excessively low.

Figure 5.8

a big share of the deficit you've created based on your current food intake, but it in no way makes it a low-carb diet. Blood sugar levels are critical to the brain and body, so your brain won't let you go too far without throwing a tantrum.

At this point, you may feel hungry, possibly weak and shaky, may be tired, and may be headachy. Since this is not a low-carb diet, this phase will be brief and is a rite of passage leading to success.

You now have reached a level of carbohydrate depletion that opens a door to significant body-fat loss. If you give in to the hunger now, you'll refill your muscle and liver glycogen as well as your bloodstream glucose (sugar), and you'll have to *start over*.

Unfortunately this is the pattern many dieters take. Three or four days go well, and then a binge sends them back to the starting block physically and mentally. What happens is they deplete and replete carb stores without much alteration in body fat. Although they really are eating well 80 percent of the time, they don't lose weight.

Average Joe Physiology

Blame Mom and Dad—A Little

Though genetics are often wrongly blamed for weight management woes, it would be a great mistake to dismiss the subject. As much as we have learned about genetics in the last generation, it is a case of "the more you learn, the more you realize you don't know." Two clear issues regarding weight-gain genetics are body-fat cell volume and hormones that control hunger. We all have a genetic range of body-fat cells that we were born with. The proliferation of these cells is greatest during the first year of life and then a second surge is possible during puberty. It is difficult to actually increase the number of body-fat cells at other times except in the case of extreme and rapid weight gain. Most fat storage is done within the number of body-fat cells already created. However, this can be a wide range, for example, 15 billion in 1 person or 250 billion in another. The sheer cell mass of the extra fat cells is significant, but more of a factor is that fat cells don't remain empty. Triglycerides can be removed and kept to a minimum, but the dynamic activity of metabolism makes it likely that small amounts of reserves will be left. This also increases the body's ability and ease of storing body fat—a major disadvantage. Multiply that by an exponentially large amount of body-fat cells, and it's easy to see how some people have "bigger frames," have "always been hefty," and have similar genetic shapes compared to parents and siblings. This isn't a life-sentence to be or remain obese, but it certainly makes it more challenging for some.

Leptin is a hormone discovered to control hunger and could be a key component in obesity and potentially a future pharmacological focus on treating it. Body-fat cells secrete leptin into the bloodstream proportionately to the amount of stored triglycerides. The hormone decreases hunger. This discovery gives credence to the "set point" theory—that our bodies have a preferred weight. If the message isn't being transmitted properly that "there is enough fat stored," a person wouldn't feel satisfied and would continue to eat. This is a very exciting area of study, but no one knows the outcome or possible side effects yet.

Diet and exercise, though, work every time.

If you stay within your macronutrient range (as indicated on Figure 5.1) through this tough-but-short phase of being moderately carb depleted, a great accomplishment takes place. Since you're not giving in to the carb cravings, your brain is forced to go to plan B. Plan B is finding an additional source of energy.

Our amazingly designed bodies will now set two things in motion that will allow for immediate and consistent fat loss. Body fat cells start doing what we want them to do! They start releasing fatty acids and glycerol, the products of stored body fat. Once in the bloodstream, some is used directly by certain types of cells for energy (lipolysis), while more gets converted into glucose. This mechanism is called gluconeogenesis, literally the creation of new glucose.

Now blood sugar levels come back up to a normal level so energy returns and hunger decreases. As a matter of fact, there's an almost euphoric rise in energy and a marked decrease in lethargy throughout the day due to the consistency in your blood sugar level. And this is real energy—not the temporary caffeine or sugar high that leaves you jittery, dazed, and then sleepy.

As long as you're consistently following the suggested food intake totals, you're now making up the majority of the caloric deficit through the mechanism of turning your body fat into new carbohydrates. The purpose of this intelligent design is so we can survive for long periods of time by accessing these calories stored in the form of body fat when necessary. By learning how to effectively take advantage of this inherent survival mechanism, you're going to lose body fat permanently and without the suffering fad diets often cause.

Another way of explaining this process is that the brain needs a constant supply of glucose in the bloodstream. To make sure glucose levels aren't too high or too low, the brain directs the pancreas to produce more glucagon (to raise blood sugar) or insulin (to store blood sugar). Fat loss or fat gain *isn't* the primary goal of the body with food; it's an indirect effect based on what hormone—glucagon or insulin—is present most often. Too many carbohydrates in one meal results in insulin being dominant. Then we're in a "storage mode." Too little carbohydrates and we're in a "retrieving mode."

Why not eliminate carbs completely? You can review chapter 2 for why carbs are an important part of a healthy diet. When too much carbohydrate is present and insulin runs rampant, we store the glucose in our liver and muscle (meaning we have to once again deplete those carbohydrate sources before burning body fat), and some of the blood glucose gets directly pulled into fat cells and stored as fat. Yo-yo dieting for sure.

One thing to keep in mind is that each gram of glycogen holds approximately three times its weight in water. A by-product of cellular metabolism is also water. The first week of decreasing your body's level of stored carbohydrates and beginning the process of losing body fat will result in a large amount of water loss. As we noted earlier, it's not uncommon to lose five to seven pounds in the first week. The second week's weight loss will be a truer reflection of how much body fat is being lost.

Experts may disagree on the methods to lose weight, but there are some things on which everyone can agree: We must cut calories, decrease fat intake, restrict carbs, and exercise. The Diet Docs' Rx does these three things while stressing whole grains, fruits, and vegetables in an amount that won't leave your glucose-hungry brain deprived. Combined with the other tools you're getting, your results can be consistent and permanent, and, at the same time, your choices can have flexibility.

Eat, Pappa! Eat!

Yes, you get to eat on the Diet Docs' plan! In fact, at times it will seem like you're eating more than you did when you were dieting in the past. You must eat enough in your optimal range to maximize your metabolism.

To lose weight effectively, you need to *stay ahead of hunger*. Eat your meals and snacks *even if you don't feel hungry*. If you allow too much time between meals or snacks, your blood sugar will drop and you will feel hungry and be tempted to binge. Don't! Plan ahead. Create new, healthy habits to replace your bad habits. Much of eating is habitual, and you'll be amazed how easy it is to replace that pink coconut marshmallow ball thing with a protein bar.

You've experienced the consequences of impulsive and unwise choices. And junk food will always be out there. It's not like you'll never get to eat any for the rest of your life. Do you recall that old Doritos commercial with Jay Leno? The tag line was something like "Eat all you want; we'll make more." Of course they will! The supply of junk food will never go away.

Decide that you will no longer continue to eat junk because you want to be healthy. Send a message to the junk food industry. There are alternatives to sugar and trans-fats and you want them!

Creating new habits will only take a matter of weeks if you focus. Do your own shopping, not relying on anyone else to take care of your responsibilities. Remember: You are becoming your own nutritionist. Study the labels. Know where the healthy food can be found in the store and which stores carry the freshest ingredients. Avoid processed foods such as crackers, chips, and cookies. Sure they taste good, but once you open a bag it's difficult to put it down.

Processed foods cause huge releases of insulin, which will instruct your body to store excess calories in your fat cells and put your pancreas under unbelievable strain. That important organ, buried deep in the middle of your abdomen, will finally say "No mas" and stop functioning properly. When that happens, you have type II (adult onset) diabetes. It's that simple.

Many people think that with our current medical technology we can cure diabetes. We do have medicines to treat the disease, but we can't cure it. And because of our increasing weight, diabetes is occurring in epidemic proportions. It's a leading cause of blindness, kidney failure, heart attacks, and even amputations. Are three sodas a day worth the loss of your leg? Practice putting good fuel in your tank, and meals will be a pleasure and an adventure instead of another opportunity for failure and the advancement of diseases.

Scott used to roll his eyes when patients told him they "didn't eat anything" yet couldn't lose weight. One of the reasons was they didn't eat enough. They basically tricked their bodies into thinking they were starving, and their bodies tried as hard as they could to hold on to the few calories they were taking in. These people needed to eat more to lose weight.

Often people mistakenly think they're not eating much. Because they're not tracking their food, they have no idea that their intake is high enough to impair fat loss. Our goal is to show you how to eat the proper amounts of the right foods to accelerate your weight loss instead of stalling or failing due to lack of knowledge or motivation.

Can't I Have Just One Piece?

Let's end this all-important chapter with the best news of the book so far. At the end of the first week (and once during every subsequent week), you get a "splurge" meal. Not a splurge *day* and not a lay-on-the-couch-moaning splurge after visiting every buffet in town.

If you're on track with your personal Diet Docs' Rx and you're losing at the pace described, you can and should have one meal per week to enjoy foods you've been avoiding. Have a couple pieces of pizza and a dessert. Have a steak, potato, and dinner roll. Eat a moderate amount and enjoy it without guilt. You'll be replacing your normal dinner and possibly a snack, so the calorie overage isn't that much—perhaps just barely over your metabolic rate.

This splurge meal accomplishes several things. First, you need that boost in food intake so your body doesn't continue in a chronic calorie deficit for too long. Second, you get a nice break from the feeling of being deprived. You may not think you need these breaks. You're tough, right? But chronic depletion can sneak up on you. Having this once-a-week "time out" makes you less prone to bingeing. You really do need it physiologically and psychologically for long-term progress.

Some nice side effects are that you get used to eating "normal" or "bad" food (however you want to describe it) without going over-board in volume, and you have the flexibility of a floating meal to use for special occasions. Plan your splurge meal for that birthday party or football game. Eat your splurge meal! If it slows your progress way down, cut your daily amount of carbs just a little to keep moving forward without cutting out this change of pace.

Your first splurge meal comes at the *end* of your first week…not tonight or tomorrow or four days from now. You can wait that long… and by then, the numbers on your scales should give you cause to celebrate your first week of weight loss!

To help you get started, at the end of this chapter are Nutrition Journal and Weekly Nutrition Log pages. Photocopy and use them to help you stay focused.

Key Points

1. Correct nutrition can raise your metabolism to help achieve weight loss.

2. The right amount of food per day is the first and most impor-tant step in achieving permanent and predictable weight loss through raising your metabolism.

3. You must follow your macronutrient totals consistently to achieve this predictable body fat loss. Take your Rx!

4. It may be necessary to adjust your macronutrient totals.

5. After two to four days, be prepared to feel hungry, tired, and possibly get headachy as your body prepares to convert body fat into glucose. Stay on course. These symptoms will only last one or two days.

6. Be patient. You're learning a lot of information. It will coalesce as you keep reading.

Nutrition Journal

Date: _____ Week: _____ Day: _____ Weight: _____

Meal	Portion Size	Food Consumed	Total Grams Per Meal			Calories
			Pro	Carb	Fat	
1						
2						
3						
4						
5						
6						
7						
Totals For Today						

Figure 5.9

Weekly Nutrition Log

Week One

Day	Protein	Carbs	Fat	Calories	Comments	Weight
1						
2						
3						
4						
5						
6						
7						
Avg.						

Week Two

Day	Protein	Carbs	Fat	Calories	Comments	Weight
1						
2						
3						
4						
5						
6						
7						
Avg.						

Week Three

Day	Protein	Carbs	Fat	Calories	Comments	Weight
1						
2						
3						
4						
5						
6						
7						
Avg.						

Figure 5.10

Weekly Nutrition Log

Week One

Day	Protein	Carbs	Fat	Calories	Comments	Weight
1						
2						
3						
4						
5						
6						
7						
Avg.						

Week Two

Day	Protein	Carbs	Fat	Calories	Comments	Weight
1						
2						
3						
4						
5						
6						
7						
Avg.						

Week Three

Day	Protein	Carbs	Fat	Calories	Comments	Weight
1						
2						
3						
4						
5						
6						
7						
Avg.						

Figure 5.10

CHAPTER 6

Meals, Power Spacing, & Other Fun Stuff

Okay, you've read the Rx chart in chapter 5 (Figure 5.1). You know your allowable portion of macronutrients for each day, right? So what do you do now?

Next up is structuring this food into daily meals and snacks for optimum results. This is a very important part of the process because you will gain or lose weight depending on how you schedule your meals. Even if you eat the right foods, you can gain weight if you don't structure your meals. There's a limit to how much food your body can effectively digest, metabolize, and absorb at one time. If you eat too much at a meal, some of that food ends up stored as new body fat.

At best, this will slow your progress; at worst, it could negate your progress. Our culture's typical way of eating promotes this pattern: skip breakfast, grab a candy bar or burger at lunch, and eat a heavy supper in the evening, followed by a trail of snacks until bedtime.

To create energy our bodies first draw dominantly from intermediate energy sources, mostly the stored glycogen in the liver and muscle. Only when most of what is stored there is used do our bodies switch in a larger way to stored body fat. So if we constantly eat larger meals, even though we stay calorically in line for the day, we have periods of time where insulin is released in high amounts, restoring our glycogen supply, which moves us out of the accelerated body fat burning mode. Not only does this style of eating promote consuming too much at one time, it also means going for long periods of time without eating, which brings up another problem.

Once the digestion, absorption, and metabolism of consumed nutrients have slowed and stopped after a meal, your body starts using stored energy. If you go too long without eating, your metabolic processes taper off to conserve energy. If you eat only a couple of large meals per day, your body converts the excess food from large meals into body fat at the same time that glycogen is being restored. During the long periods between meals, your metabolism slows down. Essentially you have created a downward spiral of storing new body fat while slowing metabolism. Furthermore, you will be prone to storing more body fat at the next meal due to the hormonal changes caused by eating a lot and then fasting. Talk about a vicious cycle!

Ironically, the act of digesting food and the subsequent increase of cellular metabolism that takes place is actually the greatest way to affect long-term calorie burning. The more times you eat, the higher your metabolism rises within your genetic limit. So don't skip your snacks. Yes, skipping a meal or snack once in a while isn't going to send your metabolism tumbling. But making this a way of life will. The biggest reason that smaller meals work better is you don't store extra body fat like you would at larger meals *and* your metabolism is increased every time you eat. If you can raise your metabolism more frequently with smaller meals and you're not storing new fat at those meals, you're in fat loss overdrive!

Power Spacing

Five to eight small meals and snacks per day is your goal. By frequently eating meals small enough that they're completely used and not stored as body fat, you keep your metabolism charged at a maximum level. Sometimes you may not be hungry at snack time, but stick to your schedule. If you skip your snack and then can't eat for another couple of hours, hunger may drive you to binge or eat something unplanned.

Power Spacing Sample	
6:00 a.m.	Breakfast
9:00 a.m.	Snack
12:00 p.m.	Lunch
3:00 p.m.	Snack
6:00 p.m.	Supper
9:00 p.m.	Small snack (optional)

Figure 6.1

Several factors make it easy to design a workable meal-spacing plan. First, divide the quantity of macronutrients logically, which isn't necessarily perfectly. Two to three meals per day should be solid, normal meals, much the same as you may currently eat except for portion size. (Food choices and meals with macronutrient ratios will be discussed in later chapters.) The remaining two to three meals per day will be smaller snacks. Schedule your meals and snacks every three to four hours.

You're probably grumbling, "I don't have time to eat that many times a day!" Scott certainly viewed this as a barrier. Can you imagine being a family practice physician and trying to find time to eat? By nine o'clock in the morning doctors are already 14 hours behind. Be honest, though. You can sip on a protein shake or stop for five minutes to grab a snack even if you're working. Here's another reason to plan ahead: Power spacing is second only to The Diet Docs' Rx (eating the right amount of the macronutrients as shown on Figure 5.1 in chapter 5) in importance if you want to achieve the safest, most efficient weight loss. For some of you, this may feel a bit clumsy at first, until you get into the habit…but it *is* critical and you *can* do it.

Your body is essentially in a constant state of metabolic storage or retrieval. Blood nutrient levels are being kept steady by the work of every system in your body. After a meal, the body is working to digest and distribute nutrients in a pattern based on priority. Processes are

Average Joe Physiology

The Dynamic Duo

Believe it or not, gaining or losing body fat is merely a symptom of a delicate balance of hormones in your body. As you now know, insulin causes glucose (carbohydrates) to be stored. Using your glucagon instigates fat loss. Insulin stores; glucagon retrieves. Insulin creates fat stores; glucagon removes stored body fat.

In a normal state of balance in the body, three times more insulin is present in the bloodstream compared to glucagon. The fact that there is a 50 million times greater amount of blood glucose than these two hormones combined shows how powerful they are in small amounts.

Subtle swings in either direction cause major metabolic changes. Imagine a teeter-totter with glucagon on one side and insulin on the other. When insulin increases above its normal levels, the body starts storing more energy than normal. If glucagon starts increasing, energy will be harvested within the body. Studies show that when carbohydrates are decreased, glucagon concentration increases. Through a cascade of events, body fat is then used as energy. When meal intervals are well-planned, sudden increases in carbohydrates, and, therefore, insulin, are easier to avoid. Over the course of a day, a week, and a month, we will spend more time with higher blood levels of glucagon compared to insulin and will lose more body fat—even with a similar overall calorie intake.

This gives us quite an edge in dieting. We're working with our bodies instead of against them.

occurring to keep the body functioning at its highest level. As critical needs are met, excess food is quickly stored. Remember, the body is built for survival. What it doesn't need now, it will store to use later. Excess fat in a meal will be stored as body fat right out of the bloodstream and excess carbohydrates will be converted into triglycerides and also stuffed into fat cells.

The bottom line is that too much food in one meal will create new body fat, based on the premise that your body will need it later. This happens constantly even to people whose weight is very stable. We store a little body fat and then use it between meals. Those of us who carry more weight than is healthy are walking reminders that we're storing more fat at those meals than we're using.

The answer isn't to wait longer between meals; the answer is to *not overeat* at meals and *stop* the storage process before it starts. This is essential because we store body fat much easier than we can use it.

Once digestion and absorption are complete after a meal and our blood sugar levels start to lower, we now have to work our way through the newly stored glycogen in the liver and the blood lipids (fat) before we start using more of the stored body fat. If we overeat, we may never get to that level of working through stored fat before we eat again and restart the process!

Conversely, if we eat meals that contain the correct amounts of protein, carbohydrates, and fat that keep our bodies functioning optimally, we increase the likelihood of not storing anything new as fat. Instead, more time is spent between meals in retrieval mode—burning stored body fat for energy. You'll soon find you're ready for that next meal even if you're not used to eating frequently. You can quickly establish a pattern of stability in your metabolism that keeps blood nutrient levels from fluctuating wildly, energy levels high, and body fat usage constant.

Should meals be exactly the same size and spaced exactly at certain intervals? If you're that obsessive compulsive, life itself has probably given you an anxiety disorder, and we don't want to add to it! You might assume there must be a perfect formula since nutrition is a science, but your daily activities, schedule, and energy expenditure create a ton of metabolic diversity.

Depending on your daily living activities and exercise, you may have different metabolic needs and hunger patterns on different days. Allow the flexibility for meals to vary in size, time, and content day to day without thinking you're failing. You'll gradually find some habits becoming mainstays and other meal and snack options may change often. By not having a rigid schedule, you'll also learn to think on your feet regarding food choices. A novel idea in this era of cookie-cutter diet books.

The Convenience Factor

Eating five to eight times a day poses a scheduling challenge for most people, just as it did with Scott. As he discovered, once you're used to this new way of eating, you'll have so much more energy that you'll never want to revert to your old meal pattern. Gone is the temporary, artificial energy brought on by sugar and caffeine. In its place is a stream of constant energy from steady blood glucose levels. Eating small, frequent meals keeps nutrients flowing into your body, which is the cornerstone of good health and weight management. Blood sugar, nitrogen (protein), and blood lipid (fat) levels all stay more uniform via small meals. Everyone has experienced lulls (and even crashes) in energy during the day. With well-spaced meals, these will disappear and be replaced with a high and steady energy level.

You can easily overcome meal scheduling challenges with good planning. Meal replacement drinks (protein shakes) and high-quality food (energy) bars are very good, convenient snack choices. Low-glycemic fruit (see chapter 2, Figure 2.5), yogurt, and many other whole-food choices are also easy to fit into your daily routine.

Even if there were such a thing as meal timing and quantity perfection, you would still have a problem sustaining that perfect schedule every day. The good news is that you don't have to. Some days are understandably going to be wild, on the run, and impossible to manage. The first thing to always consider is your ultimate goal. If you're in a hurry, don't use it as an excuse to stop for a cookie-dough milkshake because you "don't have time for anything else." It's always better to grab a healthy carb source, such as a piece of fruit, even if it causes you to be out of your macronutrient range for the day (because you may be low on protein or fat). The extra carbs won't do that much damage in that scenario. It may not be a perfect day, but it's not a diet catastrophe.

Stay well-armed with good food and plan ahead to make sure you can eat when scheduled. But when all else fails, get the best alternative you can and regroup. This is where your log book comes in handy. If you keep a running total of what you've consumed for the day, you'll make better choices on the spot. Even with no one looking over your shoulder, you'll feel rewarded, knowing you're staying on your plan even in a pinch. These small daily successes make you a confident weight-loss warrior.

Measuring Cups and Calculators

Eating the right amount of food per day and dividing that food into small meals (power spacing) are the first steps in creating your eating structure. You now know the importance of each macronutrient and some of the better choices of each. The big questions: Do I have to have the same amount of protein, carbs, and fat in each meal? Do I have to have the same ratios or proportions of nutrients in each meal?

Yes and no. To allow some flexibility, establishing a small range in each macronutrient is better than a rigid amount of food per meal or per day. Once you're locked into a "normal" eating pattern within your daily totals, you will achieve the best results if your meals represent a fairly even distribution of macronutrients throughout the day. Consuming 60 grams of carbs in one meal and only 10 in the next isn't going to cut it. You want a good ratio of nutrients in each meal to promote a stable blood sugar level, leading to stable energy and less hunger.

There are times when flexibility is not only helpful, but simply the right thing to do. For example, if you've just performed an intense workout, your next meal may include a little higher percentage of carbohydrates to refill the stored glycogen (sugar) used in the muscle tissue. If you're going to bed soon and you're hungry, it would be better to have a higher percentage of protein and less carbs. This will stimulate more growth hormone to be released at night, which can aid in recovery, rest, *and* weight loss.

You will also find that you're hungrier at specific times during the day. You may need a small meal only two hours after eating during the morning, but you can go three hours after lunch. Some meals will be larger, and some smaller. The point is that flexibility is often helpful due to schedules, is often physiologically necessary, and can help with your compliance and willingness to stay with this new eating pattern.

There is a balance between what is right nutritionally and the level you can achieve in your daily life.

Key Points

1. Too much food at one meal leads to new body fat storage.

2. Too much time between meals slows your metabolism.

3. Five to eight small meals/snacks can maximize metabolic rate and keep body-fat loss consistent.

4. Well-planned and power spaced meals lead to a steady, high energy level throughout the day.

5. Convenience is very important. Plan ahead to make sure you can eat when scheduled.

6. Keep nutrients fairly equally spaced throughout meals.

7. Allow flexibility when necessary regarding meal ratios, but stay within your nutrient totals for the day.

8. Remember power spacing!

9. Learn your body's natural hunger patterns and adjust meal spacing accordingly, allowing for some flexibility.

The Diet Docs in Action...

John's Story

I have been overweight since I was eight or nine years old. Over the years I would exercise or diet, losing anywhere from 5 to 30 pounds. Always I would put those pounds back on quickly. Soon I would give up. When I got married my wife expressed her desire for me to live a long life, so I began dieting again. I was doing great until she became pregnant with our first child. I lost focus, and shortly after our daughter was born, I had ballooned to over 300 pounds. I wasn't concerned. I rationalized that I didn't have high blood pressure, my cholesterol was okay, and I knew my wife loved me as I was (sound familiar Dr. Uloth?).

But God began to work on me. I had been facilitating a men's group that was going through *The Man God Uses* by Henry Blackaby when a thought began to recur. *John, how can you be effectively used by God if you don't take care of the body He entrusted to you? There are consequences to the neglect and sin of your indulgences, such as a tired body and even a shortened life.* But how? Diets never work for me. What is different this time? God was at work, and He was placing the people in my path to help me succeed. He answered my prayer.

I've been in a couple's small group for four years, and one of the members is Kyle. A little over a year and a half ago Kyle started going to a guy to help him lose weight and get fit. He'd heard of this guy who helped others lose the pounds. I thought, *I'll watch and see, but I'm not convinced. I mean, I have gone to "guys" before, taken pills, hit the gym, and look at me—I am big and proud of it!* Well, not really, but that's what I told myself.

The months went by and Kyle began to lose. I noticed him get smaller at each meeting and thought, *Hmmm, this seems to be working pretty well for him.* But he was working out and really into it. I wasn't ready for that! I didn't ask many questions about what he was doing. I simply watched and waited. He continued to lose until he had dropped 60 pounds and looked lean and mean. Even with his example, I still couldn't get motivated. It costs money to go to "the guy," and we were on a tight budget. Plus it would mean working out, and well, that didn't seem fun to me. Then God got my attention. I ballooned to 318 pounds. I began to labor at getting up and down to play with my 14-month-old daughter, and I couldn't keep up with my wife. Not a good sign for someone who wanted to be used by God.

continued ——➤

Then our church began to do a series on health and weight loss entitled "Body Stewardship." The class was taught by Dr. Scott Uloth and Dr. Joe Klemczewski. Wait, who? Dr. Joe? That seemed odd. Isn't that what Kyle called the guy he'd been going to? So the next meeting, I asked Kyle if he was seeing Dr. Joe Klemsooski, Klemhorsky, oh, Dr. Joe something or other. "Yes," he told me. "He's the guy."

Okay, God. I can go to this class for four Sundays for free to see what's up, but no promises! The moment either one of those guys mentions exercise everyday for an hour I am done! But you know what happened? It was amazing. They educated me. I learned that even though an ad on TV says, "Eat me! I am healthy. I am whole grain!". doesn't mean a thing. And, oh yeah, it does matter how you start your day. Furthermore, eat more meals, just not so much. They began to make me my own nutritionist. I was shown how I could become a "fat-burning machine." It all *sounded* good, but as a pessimist I wasn't convinced. The homework they gave the first week was to track what I ate—and that meant everything: carbs, fat, and protein. This was different. I had never looked at that stuff before. I thought if it was low-fat it was good for me; and aren't potatoes and corn vegetables? That's good, right? Well, not a big no, but they are not good together with a big helping of bread, fried chicken, and dumplings with a bowl of ice cream for dessert. Lots of carbs; not a lot of protein.

Fast forward to the end of the second session where I found out just how bad I was eating. I was depressed and thought, *No way can I hit the targets I should be at for my height. It's over.* I decided to e-mail Dr. Joe. He looked at my levels, and where I thought I failed he said, "You're not that far off. Make some minor adjustments, use the tips I gave you, and see." I did. One of the tips was a mentor, and well that was easy. I asked Kyle, who was more than happy to share his tips and success. I told myself, *I'll do this and see, but no exercise until I am below 290 pounds.* I didn't think I would ever get there. Guess what? I did! And now I have to exercise. Darn those promises to myself! I only did 15 minutes 3 days a week. I walked less than a mile. I continued to lose. I felt better. I advanced to jogging. One mile, two miles, then *three!* I lost 30 pounds, 50 pounds, 75 pounds! I am now at over 120 pounds lost and counting. I'm in clothes I didn't even know existed in high school. I set a goal of 195 pounds by April 2008—a goal I thought I would never come close to. I am now at 196 pounds in February.

continued ——➤

The Diet Docs' program has changed my life. I'm feeling great and have more confidence. My back doesn't hurt, and I can play with my daughter and newborn son without getting out of breath.

This is my desire for you: to truly be blessed as I have with this program, for you to decide to give it a try. Maybe God wants you to take a leap of faith as I did so He can come through in a big way as He did for me. This is all for His glory. He was the reason, and he has used Dr. Uloth and Dr. Joe to change me and give me the chance to be used for His glory a little longer.

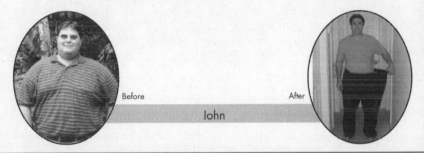

Before   After

John

CHAPTER 7

Use It or Lose It!

See Scott Run

Okay, Maggot! Get in here! Prepare to eat tofu, tree bark, and birdseed. And you'll like it! Prepare for pain and lots of it, Mr. Chicken-Wings-for-Arms. Now drop and give me 20 or until you puke, whichever comes last, you soda-guzzling, cheese curl-munching pud!"

That's what I expected to hear the first time I walked into Club Fitness Zone, the first serious gym I'd gone to since college. I expected to find a bunch of jocks waiting to give me a wedgie, or even worse, having to help me dislodge from a piece of exercise equipment I had no idea how to use. ("Hey, the new guy got himself caught in the Hamstring Strangulator again. What a weenie. It's your turn to get him out.")

What I found, however, was a group of people much like me who were more concerned with camaraderie and their own health than watching someone else mess up. The local sheriff, attorneys, teachers, business persons, and work-at-home moms were all there improving their health.

Many of them had similar stories of how they overcame the weight-loss demons. One gentleman had lowered his triglycerides from 900 to 90. A middle-aged woman had lost 60 pounds and kept it off. Another person had rehabbed from debilitating back problems. Each person had a different story, but each one was clear about the goals he or she wanted to achieve.

I learned an important lesson from these people: *Don't be intimidated.* Whether you decide to work out at a local gym or exercise at home where family may make fun of your Spandex, just relax and make your time enjoyable. Forget how you look. Forget how clumsy you are at first. The important thing is getting started. You'll make mistakes and feel awkward, but that's okay. Fitness is a marathon, not a sprint.

Do I Have To?

The gym Scott mentions was a small facility I (Joe) bought more than a decade ago. I steadily expanded services with nutrition programs and personal trainers as I stumbled around seeking a business identity. My desire was to have a place for anyone with any goal I could help them reach. If you wanted a nutrition consultation, or some personal training, or a comprehensive fitness program, or simply a gym membership, I had you covered.

One thing I learned early is that a successful client was my greatest marketing asset. I didn't have a clue about marketing and knew even less about sales, but I poured my guts out to help clients succeed who were willing to jump on board. I constantly worked to improve, restructure, and reinvent our programs to increase client success.

At one point I had to make a hard decision. Those referred to me for weight loss would often choose a single consultation to develop a nutrition program and then be gone. Others would opt for follow-up nutrition work to help implement their program. Still others would sign on for nutrition and also lock in to a series of personal training sessions that often led to a regular schedule. Guess which group blew everyone else away in consistent and permanent results?

Once I realized those who errantly thought "buying a program" from me and trying to implement it on their own was a magic bullet, I felt a moral obligation to revamp my business and only offer what works. So instead of operating from a volume approach, where the emphasis was being accessible by price, I swallowed hard and designed an eight-week program that included nutrition and training. I loved the concept of having clients for that long of a period to help them cement their newfound knowledge with experience and launch them toward their goal.

Most people were glad to commit to such an all-inclusive plan once they knew victory was assured. Today I still have that program, but now it's six months long and includes an initial evaluation/consultation, a follow-up nutrition meeting, a fitness consultation, a series of training sessions to implement a fitness program with an exercise physiologist, a meeting with a staff counselor, classes on a variety of topics, and unlimited e-mail support with an online nutrition tracking system for monitoring, feedback, and necessary adjustments.

Two components of the program stand out in a big way. The first is that my staff's ongoing contact keeps clients grounded and moving forward. To that same end, Scott and I have designed the program in this book the same way—one step at a time, one day at a time, and one week at a time. The other component is that those who participate in a fitness program along with the nutritional changes recommended are creating a successful synergy of nutrition and exercise. The clients' marked improvement in energy levels and their almost immediate results were impossible to ignore. Success begets success.

One thing we always tell new clients is, "If there's anything you need us to do—an extra follow-up meeting, specific health questions or assistance, anything at all—just *ask*. If you're serious about your health and your goal, we're going to do anything it takes to help you." Now we're asking you the same question: Are you willing to do anything it takes to help yourself? Are you reading this book because you are already committed to making a change? If so, nothing will stop you from succeeding!

Rock-Hard Abs in Seven Seconds a Week

Hi! Sammy Slick here with the revolutionary new Six-Pack-Abs-in-Seven-Seconds-a-Week System! This amazing technique has been a protected secret in an ancient tribe of albino ship builders in the mountains of Norway for 32 centuries! Known for their sculpted physiques, this obscure sect successfully sheltered their clandestine system—until now! Recently excommunicated for allowing his body fat to elevate above 5 percent, a seventeenth-generation ab-master has given us an exclusive tell-all interview. For only three payments of $39.95 you can learn how a simple breathing technique will transform your body in just seven seconds a week. That's right! *Seven seconds a week!* Use it while watching your favorite sitcom, standing in line at your favorite fast-food restaurant, or even while sleeping. But that's not all! Order now and we'll include the never-seen-before secret tribal isometric granite-glute contraction routine absolutely free. Both systems can be employed simultaneously, giving you a whole body workout without breaking a sweat!

(Results may vary. Limited to customers genetically tested to have limited body-fat cells and even fewer brain cells. Guarantee void if the system is not used with the zero-calorie diet included.)

Come on, tell the truth. You've been tempted by the outlandish promises on these infomercials for expensive exercise equipment, haven't you? Well, we can't promise that weight loss is quite *that* easy, but fitness doesn't have to be hard. We even dare to say you might enjoy it. In the rest of the chapter we will be focusing on the benefits and options and help you understand why exercise needs to be a regular part of your weight-loss plan.

Jack LaLanne Isn't an Exception

Joe recently heard longtime fitness advocate (back when fitness wasn't cool) Jack LaLanne give a lecture. He is quite exceptional, but he's not a mutant who defies the laws of aging. Now in his mid-nineties, Jack says he hasn't eaten a dessert since the 1920s, after overcoming childhood sicknesses with nutrition and exercise. (Aren't you glad The Diet Docs' mantra is "flexibility"?) If you were to study most research results and exercise physiology textbooks, you would see that what is claimed in terms of health and longevity is being lived out by this fitness pioneer.

On his seventieth birthday Jack swam a mile and a half while pulling 70 boats with 70 people aboard. Did we mention he did it with his hands and feet handcuffed? At 70 years old! *Exceptional.* Yes, exceptional, but physical prowess is accessible to people who want to spend as much time on their health as they do watching Bill O'Reilly not spin the news. The evidence is clear that God has designed our bodies to move and a certain amount of physical work is necessary for it to work...and work well. When that principle is lived out faithfully...well, you may end up living a life like Jack has!

Research shows that those who exercise have better cognition and extended brain health. Exercise also increases bone mass and decreases the risk of osteoporosis. And it's not news that exercise significantly decreases heart disease and stroke factors. Positive effects are exerted on blood sugar metabolism as well. Further, exercise decreases the risk of arthritis and other degenerative conditions. As for cancer, exercising regularly from childhood on may result in significant decreases of cancer incidences. Increased oxygen and blood flow from exercise are primary reasons for the decreased risk.

Long ago Joe sat in an exercise physiology class in physical therapy school. He says he can still hear his professor explain the vascular benefits of exercise. The professor had an accent like Arnold Schwarzenegger, and that made it more fun to listen. One particular class he put a videotape into the VCR and for a few seconds there was nothing but a blank screen. Then a lone, white blip flittered across the screen horizontally. Then another in a different spot. Then another. Then more. The blips increased in frequency and latitude until the screen was filled with dots screeching across the screen from left to right. The Austrian-sounding educator excitedly grinned as he explained that the class was watching red blood cells in the thigh of a mouse at rest initially and then on a wheel. At rest the small capillaries in our bodies that are big enough to only carry red blood cells in single-file lines (sometimes folded in half) only receive enough oxygen to keep the tissue and cells alive. But when the heart is pumping more blood through the body, more oxygen and nutrients get to the deepest recesses of our bodies and toxic waste is removed much faster. Cancer cells don't like oxygen; healthy cells do.

Um…I Bought a Diet Book

In addition to the health benefits mentioned, several good things happen in an overall weight-loss plan when you include exercise. The most obvious is that you're burning calories. When you do the math, you find that cutting 500 calories from your daily metabolic needs (a pound of body fat being roughly 3,500 calories) means a loss of about a pound per week. Eventually, however, as your store of energy available from fat diminishes, your pace may slow. Couple that with perhaps having a genetically slow metabolism, and you may feel you're moving too slowly toward your goal. The *great* news is that exercise can double your speed on the other side of the energy ledger: calorie expenditure.

Many people also find that exercise *decreases* hunger. A client recently told Joe she was moving her daily cardiovascular exercise to mid-afternoon. He told her it was a great idea because he knew she had also mentioned becoming a little hungry at that time of the day. Sure enough, due to the changes that occur between the brain, muscular system, and digestive system going from rest to activity, she reported that her afternoon hunger was avoided by the change in her routine.

When we ask a new client what his or her goals are, feeling better usually comes right after weight loss. Sometimes it's even the primary plea. Nothing will make you feel better than exercise. That's a strong

Average Joe Physiology

Calories in ➤ Calories OUT

After exercise, your body continues to use an increased amount of calories for approximately 90 minutes. The level of energy expenditure—the intensity of the activity—dictates how many calories you're using above your basal metabolic rate and how long after training you will see the amplified calorie burn continue. Per 30 minute session, here is where various activities rate:

Exercise	Calories used by 150-pound person	Calories used by 200-pound person
Stationary bicycling	245	310
Housecleaning	120	155
Ballroom dancing	190	245
Golf	140	180
Jogging	245	310
Race walking	275	320
Running 6 mph (10-minute mile)	345	440
Swimming laps (light effort)	275	355
Walking 3 mph	120	155
Weight lifting (vigorous effort)	205	265

As you can see, a little exercise can go a long way calorically in helping you reach your weight-loss goal. Multiply the calorie expenditure by the number of days you perform the activity per week and then by the number of months you are in weight-loss mode. That's a lot of calories being used!

statement, we know. And we stand by it. Research proves it. One neuroscientist Joe was recently listening to reported that as we get older exercise has a better effect on depression than antidepressants. (But please, don't stop taking your medications in favor of the elliptical machine without your physician's permission.)

If you ask people who know Joe, they may tell you that, as a bit of an oddity for a professional bodybuilder, he likes to run. The truth is he doesn't really like to run. It's never on the top of his list of things to do. He can easily find reasons to push it off his schedule, and he jokes that he's about the worst distance guy you'll find on the track. But he likes the way he feels every second of the day when he includes running in his routine. He explains that he feels lighter, stronger, more agile, and truly experiences an improvement in his brain energy and cardiovascular health.

Joe's feeble attempts to emulate real runners also mean he's burning more calories. That's a huge motivator! And that motivation carries over. The invested time and effort motivate him to be even more consistent with food intake. He's not about to spend all that time on a treadmill and then go home and grab a bag of Oreos!

Dude, I Hate the Gym

We're not going to tell you that running, doing crunches, and lifting mega-amounts of weight in a gym every day are the only ways to stay fit, but we agree with all the research that your best overall fitness and weight loss results will come from including regular exercise. For some, the place to start may be simply walking around the block. Others will find that ballroom dancing and other recreational hobbies are perfect workouts. When your heart beats faster—it *is* a muscle, you know—it gets stronger. As the heart gets stronger, every heartbeat will push more blood per stroke through the body and do it more efficiently. As your body's need for oxygen is increased due to the exercise, your lungs get better at replacing carbon dioxide with oxygen. Even at rest, your now-stronger heart and more-capable lungs keep your body cleaner and better supplied with oxygen with less cost in terms of body system stress. Can you say "anti-aging"? How about "feeling awesome"? Being healthy and feeling great is well worth the effort.

Remember our hypothetical question to clients earlier? Are you willing to do whatever it takes to succeed? Once you can easily walk once around the block safely, make it *two* laps.

If your knees are healthy and you have good shoes, dare to lightly jog for 20 feet each lap. Progressing to new levels of physical activity can be fun and should make you feel better than you knew God designed you to feel.

Caution: Before starting any exercise program, consult your doctor regarding your fitness level and any suggested restrictions. This book does not and should not take the place of medical advice.

Recommendations

Joe's facility now schedules new clients for a fitness consultation with a staff exercise physiologist for a handful of reasons. We want to assess any health or orthopedic risks, get to know the clients' fitness goals, discuss options, design plans that fit their goals, and teach them how to safely execute the plan. We can't recommend anything less to you. If you can do so, find a good personal trainer, preferably one with a degree in a physical science field. He or she can help you design a plan similar to the ones we create.

If you're beyond walking your dog and calling it a workout and you're looking for something to really make a difference in your health, let's get down to business. Two things we know about fitness conclusively we've already outlined: keeping your heart and lungs strong is the best way to prevent cardiovascular disease and enjoy the best benefits of fitness. The second is that Joe's work as a physical therapist has confirmed that most of the musculoskeletal pain and degeneration we encounter as we age can be avoided. The strength and flexibility gained by moderate, consistent resistance training produces staggering results in our bodies' abilities to function normally and pain-free.

Cardiovascular Rx

How much exercise do you need? For now, let's just set a goal of performing 30 minutes of cardiovascular work, 3 times a week.

At that level you'll be at what many health professionals consider the entry point to better health. In recent years our obesity-ridden culture has prompted experts to raise the bar to one hour of physical activity per day. That's a goal. For now, we'll break exercise down into beginner, intermediate, and advanced levels.

Beginners

Definition: If you engage in no physical activity at this time, start at this level.

Program: Begin a walking program with a determined time or distance interval. For example, you might start by walking 10 minutes each day and increase it by 5 minutes each week. If walking is not your thing, choose any cardiovascular activity, but make sure you keep progressing slowly.

Intermediates

Definition: If you sporadically work out or participate in recreational activities, consider beginning here.

Program: You may not be able to begin at 30 minutes per session, but build up to an activity where 70 to 80 percent of your maximum heart rate (220 minus your age multiplied by .70 to .80) is held constant for 30 minutes, 2 to 3 times per week. It could be walking, light jogging, or working out on your favorite cardiovascular equipment (rowing machine perhaps?).

Advanced

Definition: If you work out regularly already and consider yourself active, it's time to move up to the big leagues.

Program: If you already enjoy training or want the benefits of advanced fitness, let's talk about intensity versus volume. The 400 meter sprint, the mile, and the marathon are drastically different events. They place different demands on the body. Those of us who want the best results should consider steady, moderate cardiovascular exercise but also stepping it up to athletic levels. Your baseline cardiovascular health should be seen as consistent work done over time. A pace similar to that described in the intermediate level is a great place to start and work toward 30 to 40 minute sessions 3 to 5 times per week. (Three if you're including a good amount of resistance exercise and 4 to 5 if you love cardio.) Once you feel ready to progress, take 1 or 2 of your sessions and start adding higher-intensity interval work. This could be a walk/jog combination, a jog/sprint or walk/sprint pace, or simply performing a stronger-paced workout for a shorter · amount of time. The goal is to strengthen your cardiovascular system in more of an anaerobic fashion to complement your growing aerobic base. It's a good idea to do some cross-training as well. Doing the same thing all the time can lead to cumulative trauma issues and boredom.

Resistance Training Rx

As a rookie orthopedic physical therapist Joe was amazed how fast patients improved with the practice of minor tasks and therapeutic exercises. Like many, he had been conditioned in the gym to obliterate a muscle group and then give it days and days to recover. But now he was often prescribing a set of the exercises for a patient to do 2 or 3 times per day.

Even though the same muscles were worked that often, the rehabilitation sped along, and soon we were able to increase resistance, functionality, and difficulty. With the increased involvement of a muscle per session, the patient would then have to allow for more rest time. The more the body was asked to do and the higher the level of training, the less frequency was needed but more recovery time was required. In other words, start slow, let your body become conditioned, use simplicity, and as you progress you can more safely and effectively train for even greater results.

Beginners

Definition: If you have never lifted weights and don't currently engage in any structured workout program, start here.

Program: Consider allowing a professional to help you design a program. I suggest a series of floor exercises you can easily do in your living room. Start with the trunk of your body and move outward. Crunches for your abdominals, various stretches for your entire body, and some targeted exercises can put you on a path of conditioning for higher-level work. You may quickly progress to specialized DVD programs.

Intermediates

Definition: If you have worked out in the past or participate in recreational activities or sports, plug in here.

Program: Exercises similar to the beginners' can be duplicated with more advanced techniques, especially with equipment in a health club. Consider a beginning level of training that a personal trainer can map out for you in a 2- or 3-day per week program. Slowly increase intensity and resistance, but be sure to keep your form perfect to stay safe.

Advanced

Definition: For those who work out already, even if sporadically, this is where you can get the best of both worlds. You may need to take yourself through an intermediate level of work for a couple of weeks to make sure you're conditioned for progress. The advanced level is where you want to train 2 or 3 days per week (maybe even 4 or 5 if you only perform a couple of bouts of cardiovascular work each week).

Program: Once again, since you're possibly jumping into unfamiliar waters, it would be wise to meet with a professional for program design and instruction. However, there are countless books, magazines, DVDs, and websites to keep you trying new workouts for the rest of your life. I often recommend a minimum weight training program to include an "upper body day" and a "lower body day." It would be difficult to effectively train every muscle group in one session, thus the split. Even if you train some upper and lower body muscle groups each of the two days, you'll find you can accomplish a great deal in those workouts. A progression from there would be to divide your body into 3 or even 4 workouts and specialize more per workout. This is more a bodybuilding style of training, which isn't a bad configuration at all even if maximum muscle isn't your goal. It gives you a chance to experiment more, add variety, and work a little deeper into each muscle group.

Lifelong Functional Athletes

Someday soon Joe notes that his training will have a more general objective. He already considers himself a lifelong athlete who just happens to be a pro bodybuilder. He regularly plays organized basketball and can (most times) beat his son who's three inches taller than he is. He plays baseball aggressively with his boys. He runs with more than a casual interest. Joe plans on enjoying sports and training as long as God holds his body together. But don't let my bent on weight training make you think that is what fitness is all about. We both believe its value is immense, but it's more important for you to choose something you'll stick with. Set aside time to get involved with as many activities as you enjoy. You may not only have more fun, but you'll keep yourself functionally fit.

Key Points

1. Decide that your health is worth the time investment.

2. Work on cardiovascular and musculoskeletal progress.

3. Hire a professional to help design and instruct your fitness program.

4. Be patient and enjoy your progress—it can be a very enriching part of your life.

5. If you venture into a gym, be very careful around the Hamstring Strangulator!

The Diet Docs in Action...

Julie's Story

You've probably heard a lot of successful dieters say, "If I can lose weight on this diet, anyone can!" But in the case of The Diet Docs' plan, it really is true!

I had all the normal excuses for not being able to lose weight. I was over 40, had an autoimmune disorder that affected my joints, many other medical conditions, and a sluggish metabolism. Some doctors even suggested I just be satisfied with maintaining my current weight. But at 5'4" and 260 pounds, my blood pressure, blood sugar, and cholesterol were at life-threatening levels. I started on a diet program from a popular diet book and made some progress. It wasn't specific enough to help me when I "got stuck." I started regaining the weight without any idea how to reverse it. By June 2003 I was completely convinced that no diet would ever help me.

I called Dr. Joe, we decided to meet, and the rest is history.

As of October 2005, I have lost over 120 pounds and am close to my goal—weighing 130 pounds after losing 130 pounds. My latest cholesterol test (nonfasting) was 178, compared to totals in the 220s before. My blood sugar is within normal levels, and I hope to be free of all blood pressure medicines in the next few months. My joint problems have all but disappeared, along with my other health problems. No one recognizes the "old me," and I have no intention of going back there.

So what makes The Diet Docs' diet and exercise plan different? For one thing, you don't start eating special foods that help you lose weight as long as you're on them...but let you regain your weight once you return to normal eating. You start by gaining an awareness of the protein, fat, and carbohydrate balances in the foods you currently eat. It was a huge wakeup call for me—mainly the carbohydrates. I had no idea I was eating so many carbs in a day. Just understanding that problem started me down the road to better eating. The Diet Docs want you to understand the importance of looking at the foods you normally eat. I was able to look for the foods I liked, find out how to moderate them, or substitute for them, and design my own plan for diet success. I put the counts of the foods I normally ate into an Excel spreadsheet. I still carried the "food

continued →

count" book with me so I could calculate the values for new foods. If you can control the portions and fit the counts into your daily diet, no food is completely off limits. The *Diet Docs'* plan lets you take ownership of your own diet. With my busy schedule, I frequently ate in restaurants and have still been successful.

Joe also helped me understand the importance of not only aerobic but also strength exercises. He's helped guide me to an effective training program. I'm still perfecting that part! I am not a bodybuilder or an athletic person. I have trouble with coordination (walking and chewing gum!). I always thought my lack of skills would hamper my effectiveness with exercise. Not true.

I'm still not coordinated, I'm still not a bodybuilder, but I am getting to be a thinner, fitter person thanks to this plan. I'm a normal, everyday person. Believe me, if I can do it, so can you!

Does the plan work? You can probably tell from my before and after photos the answer is yes! All I can say is I used to be a size 22 and now I'm a size 4. How many 46 year olds weigh what they did at age 18 after spending years and years well over 200 pounds? It's safe to say that reading the book and following Dr. Joe's advice changed my life forever. I now have the specific tools to keep this up and to help myself recover from those inevitable holiday relapses. I can't thank him enough. But I can encourage all of you—it's never too late, and you can do it!

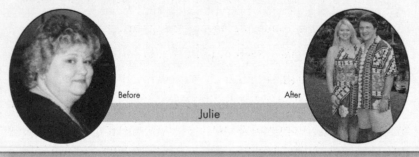

Before   After

Julie

CHAPTER 8

The Psychology of Success

Okay, here comes the all-important motivational chapter. In chapter one we identified the three keys to effective weight loss:

1. Eat the right foods to help your body burn stored fat.

2. Add appropriate exercises to further boost weight loss.

3. Stay motivated.

In previous chapters you've discovered the importance of the first two elements for permanent weight loss. Now we want to spend some time on the third aspect: getting—and staying—motivated.

When a client leaves Joe's office for the first time, he can usually predict their success with great accuracy. People who fail are those who have been given the best and most accurate information but won't apply it. Clients who take the initiative and put our program to work seldom fail. In fact, it's hard to not guarantee success to everyone because success is *possible* if the program is followed.

The Power of Patience

Let's get one thing straight as you begin. Losing weight will be work. There is no way around that. However, with a good program like this one, it isn't an overwhelming amount of work. Is anything worthwhile ever very easy? Of course not. Permanent weight loss is a lifelong commitment...and it requires patience. Nothing sends Scott from zero to crazy faster than when he's talking to a patient about diet and exercise and he gets a dismissive wave of a hand and the person says, "I already know what I need to do. I just need to do it." Be willing to take in information. You might learn something new or discover a way to do something better.

Losing weight is an incremental process. And anything that changes incrementally requires patience to bring about the desired reward. Though an age-old adage, you didn't gain your excess baggage overnight so you shouldn't expect to lose it overnight. Every legitimate study says that safe weight loss is one to two pounds per week, max. If you have 50 to 60 pounds to lose, you must accept it will take 6 or more months to lose the weight safely. Don't give up after 90 days. Keep on keeping on. You will probably hit plateaus that may take several weeks to break through. In the process of his weight loss, Scott hit two plateaus. One took three weeks to break through and the other took four. Stick with it and you will smash through too.

Motivation for those who want to lose weight is comprised of commitment plus patience. That's the equation: Commitment + patience = weight loss.

Girls (and Boys) Just Want to Have Fun

Let's face it: Food is neither illegal nor immoral, at least at this point anyway. In fact, food can be fun. We enjoy eating food that can significantly shorten our life spans. But here's the good news: As you commit to change, your tastes in food will change too. What once caused you to drool with anticipation will soon become much easier to resist.

For instance, as you decrease your carbohydrate intake, you will notice that high-sugar foods won't taste as good. Ex-smokers say the same about cigarettes. It doesn't mean they don't want one, but they can use that change in taste to their advantage the same way you can with high-sugar foods. *Do not force* yourself to learn to like those high-sugar foods again. The loss of that pleasure may be a little disappointing at first, but you can replace that sadness with the wonderful feelings of confidence and athleticism that will allow you to enjoy other areas of life that aren't food related.

We'll give you an example. Previously Scott would go to parties and as soon as he entered the gathering he was thinking about where the buffet table was located, when the meal would be served, and worrying that if he was at the end of the line there wouldn't be enough to eat. Now Scott can spend time with loved ones and friends and focus on catching up on their lives and sharing laughs and good times instead of worrying about food. Now he doesn't mind being at the back of the line.

Also, you will notice that high-fat or high-sugar foods will hurt your stomach when you aren't used to them. Learn that feeling because your body is telling you something. Listen to it! In fact, you will enjoy certain foods more since you won't be eating them as often. You'll get a greater sense of satisfaction during your "splurge meal" knowing you sacrificed and truly earned it.

Staying motivated doesn't mean you grit your teeth and resign yourself to suffering loss for the rest of your life.

Well, Excuuuuuse Me!

As you become more motivated and stay motivated, it will be important that you not accept excuses or rationalizations from yourself. Both of those will eat away at your motivation for long-term change. We're not talking about slip-ups or mistakes because even the most dedicated of us will have bad days. We're talking about letting that one bad meal turn into a bad day or week or…worse.

We'll deal more fully with some common excuses in chapter 11, but for right now let's just admit that the road to staying motivated

Average Joe Physiology

Stress Eating Is the Real Deal

You've heard the commercials for cortisol-reducing supplements: "Block the hormone that traps unwanted fat around your stomach..." We're not sure if the supplements can do much to stop your adrenal glands from producing cortisol, but a valid point is raised. Many of us admittedly are "stress eaters" or "emotional eaters." There is a very good reason. Under stress (and your brain doesn't care if it's from being chased by a grizzly bear, facing deadlines at work, or watching the nightly news) your body goes into "fight or flight" response. Your heart rate increases, blood is shunted to your muscles for action, and stored carbohydrates (glycogen) are diverted from your liver and muscle into your bloodstream for the anticipated energy needs.

As the process slows, assuming you didn't get caught by the bear or your boss, that extra blood glucose gets stored as abdominal fat. It is directed mainly to your middle because only there can it be mobilized rapidly again for conversion to glucose. Your body is thinking ahead—for survival. The problem is we're getting more and more chronic daily stress and we're not using the released energy.

The storage of the new fat deposits signal the brain to shut off the stress response, and the next phase of fight or flight is launched: operation refuel. The hard-wired expectancy of the nervous system is that after a stressful situation, energy has to be replaced. Waves of cravings follow as part of the let-down from stress. Cortisol causes direct abdominal fat storage and intense carbohydrate cravings.

(A side note: Many researchers link antidepressant drugs to weight gain for this reason. Apparently, we get locked into this step that involves bringing stress levels down when we take these medications.)

Stress must be met head-on with preparedness. When our daily lives create turmoil and intense hunger follows, we can combat it by relaxing, performing breathing exercises, walking away from the situation, drinking a glass of water, and so forth. This is to literally buy time and direct our brain to de-escalate the situation. If we find ourselves reaching for food, we need to recognize the situation at hand and make sure it doesn't lead to a binge. With this information, we don't have to be dragged under the tow of this hormone; we can stay on top with planning.

is filled with land mines that can derail you if you're not careful to avoid them. We've heard all the excuses for the loss of motivation and have experienced many of them ourselves…but we dealt with them quickly and got back on track…and you can too. Some of the most common excuses are rationalizations such as…

- I'm not really all that bad. Look at _____. He (or she) weighs more than I do and he (she) is happy.

- I don't have the right metabolism for losing weight.

- My parents were overweight so my problem must be entirely genetic.

- People need to accept me the way I am.

- I'm too busy.

- I deserve to eat what I want, when I want.

- I know what I need to do. I don't need to follow a plan.

Are You Looking at *Me*?

You must willingly forego making such excuses and accept responsibility for your dietary and exercise choices. You're not powerless over yourself, you really aren't.

You can do this program and do it beginning right now.

It took Scott forever to get started because he believed 50 pounds was too big a wall to climb. However, after he started it was the consistent choices every day that allowed him to lose 60 pounds. All of a sudden minus 50 was here and past—and it took less than 6 months! It wasn't like he'd climbed Mt. Everest, although before he started he thought it would be like that. Why did Scott wait so long? Fear of failure. Don't *you* wait. Start today!

Losing weight, even if it's 100 pounds or more, is definitely within the realm of your capability. You can do it! You are just making a bunch of fat cells get smaller. You are creating discipline and exerting the control you forgot you had. You can't control other people or external circumstances, but you can control you. You are in charge...no matter how bossy your body tries to be. You can reach for a pint of Häagean-Dazs or that lovely Granny Smith apple—it's always your choice.

Staying Motivated

You are probably motivated to begin the Diet Docs' Rx, but are you wondering if you can *stay* motivated for the long haul? *We* know you can, but *you* need to know you can. On the next page are some valuable tips that have worked for us and for others to help stay the course. These tips, along with an understanding of the pitfalls and obstacles discussed in chapter 11 will help you.

Perhaps one of the best motivators is to simply begin. The sooner you start, the sooner the elation of watching the pounds fall off!

Start Here, Start Now

In a notebook, start recording your food intake beginning today. Waiting until tomorrow might help you procrastinate to next week; next week will lead you to failure, and you may just throw away this chance to gain total control over food, your health, and your physique. So start today! Record everything you eat for a day or two as you make some small changes based on this book.

Start fine-tuning your nutrition by implementing your personal Diet Docs' Rx: choosing better foods, improving your meal spacing, concentrating on meal ratios, and adding some exercise. Before you know it, you'll be feeling better than you thought possible! You'll be losing weight and well on your way to becoming your own expert nutritionist.

In your daily journal, include a portion for writing down what you did to move your body. Keep on journaling one day at a time. Your written record will help you stay on track as you watch the pounds come off.

The Diet Docs' Tips for Staying Motivated

1. Find a partner to join you in your journey. Remember the Diet Docs' Rx can be tailored to his or her needs as well. Sharing with a friend can help you remember why you started the diet. Consider the diet a small group activity.

2. Make a habit of entering in your journal how you feel when you reach certain goals. During stressful times, go back and reread those sections and give yourself a pat on the back. Realize how far you've come.

3. Be creative. Discover recipes that delight your taste buds and further your goals. Start your own cookbook.

4. Set a goal—run a mile, walk (don't ride!) nine holes of golf, hike a mountain trail, chase your kids (or your spouse). Sometimes you need a tangible endpoint to stay motivated.

5. You are developing a recipe for success. If you haven't already cleaned out your pantry or fridge of the extra junk food, get rid of it. Out of sight, out of mind.

6. Really enjoy your splurge meal. Don't feel guilty. You've earned it by your hard work. (See how much fun Sunday dinner at the in-laws can be!)

7. Look at old photos or your old cholesterol level to remind yourself why you are doing this.

8. Give your old clothes to charity. Nothing will motivate faster than a new wardrobe or the realization that you can't go back once you've given the garments away.

9. Use your new health/energy to serve God and help others. Do a little something to take yourself out of your comfort zone.

10. Learn more. Read more about nutrition, exercise, and health-related fields from reliable sources. Be passionate about what you do.

11. Pray. Especially when you are weak, remember Philippians 4:13, 1 Corinthians 6:19-20, and Romans 12:1-2. God is not here to make you feel sad or inadequate; He is here to encourage you!

Key Points

1. Start right now!

2. Document meticulously.

3. Consistency, consistency, consistency.

4. It doesn't matter how many times you fall down, only how many times you get back up!

5. You're in this for life so be patient and enjoy the trip.

6. Prepare your mind for battle; prepare to win!

CHAPTER 9

Your First 6 Weeks

Many of Joe's clients have attended one of his lectures or met with him for a consultation and then received a copy of this material. Later they experienced the "Eureka!" moment when they were able to connect the dots of sound nutrition and get what they must do to enjoy permanent weight loss.

Rarely do clients leave without thinking they've found the missing link. They're excited to begin their new program. But they also start feeling overwhelmed by the sheer volume of new information. We want to make this process as easy as possible for you. So the following six-week start will help you process the information you've found in these pages into your eating habits one bite and step at a time. Following this six-week program has become as close to a 100 percent guarantee for your success as anything we've ever seen.

So let's get started!

Day 1...*Today*

As you start The Diet Docs' Rx, take a little time to be by yourself. Totally no distractions. Turn the television off, put the kids in bed, and find the remote for your spouse so you have a few minutes of total privacy. Think about *why* you want to lose weight and get in shape. Put down all the reasons on paper (not in your notebook). Also jot down your personal strengths and weaknesses. What were your dieting failures in the past? What led to dieting collapses? Do this in one day. Don't let this self-analysis drag on and lead to paralysis.

Now take those pages and shred them. That's right. Rip them up and dance on top of them. Laugh, cry, or spit if you need to, but tear them up. Don't tape them up on your mirror for motivation. Your memory already knows what you did right and wrong in the past. That was then, this is now. You are not a loser or a failure because of past problems. You are now a student of nutrition, and few students ever get 100 percent on every test. At the end of this course, you will be a lot smarter (and lighter) than when you started. Whether you are in denial or rationalization mode, you simply need to be honest with yourself, acknowledge that fact, and move forward.

If you truly can't leave the baggage behind, get help for your mind as well as your body and see a counselor. The baggy clothes and the candy bar stuffed behind the flour canister aren't fooling anyone. And how much does food really comfort you when you're staring at the results in the mirror and riding the guilt and shame train?

The biggest reason to understand nutrition and exercise is your health. Food is an "acceptable drug," but it can be a very destructive coping mechanism. It's that simple. Food will kill you just as dead as drugs, alcohol, and tobacco. Face it.

Overeating is that straightforward, and it never needs to get any more complicated than that. Looking better, playing more with your kids, or impressing a new coworker at the office are all nice by-products of being in shape, but they are secondary to staying healthy and living a longer, more enjoyable life.

Good health—and not just looking good—needs to be a big part of your goal. So only focus on one goal. Say this to yourself and mean it: *I want to learn about nutrition and exercise to improve my health for the rest of my life.*

We know you'll enjoy and revel in how you look when you're leaner and people start saying, "Hey! Are you working out? You look so much younger!" We want to make sure you're grounded in the long-term "why"of your metabolic transformation.

Week 1

Week 1 has a single focus: Get familiar with the charting system and begin tracking your food intake. This week may be frustrating as you start measuring food, planning meals, and calculating nutrients for journaling. The rare person who fails often stops here. If you're committed to your goals, you'll survive this step and go on to success. Take this week very seriously, and you'll understand why it's the most critical.

Once you go through the learning process of tracking your food, you'll have a databank of nutritional information memorized without even trying. As you look up foods, read nutrition fact panels, scour menus, and record your intake, you'll be amazed how easy it becomes.

At the end of the first week, you should be getting into your personal Rx ranges consistently. The first couple days will be hit and miss; don't expect to be perfect. This week is a learning process to help you understand the documentation and get used to what those suggested protein, carbohydrate, and fat intake ranges mean in terms of real food. It's one thing to see numbers on paper and another to translate them into meals.

It may be a good idea to keep your personal Diet Docs' Rx card in your pocket or in your nutrition journal (see chapter 5, Figures 5.2, 5.9, 5.10). Jot down the food counts for meals you frequently eat in the front of your journal. That way you don't have to calculate them over and over and can make faster food decisions.

At the end of chapter 5 there is a sample daily food chart and a six-week "at-a-glance" spreadsheet. Remember to record the all-important daily food, amounts, and times on this form or something similar. This will help you keep a running tally and plan for the rest of the day. The weekly chart is a great tool to study trends and zero in on what levels of food intake allow for different weight-loss numbers. Without this objectivity, it's almost impossible to learn what you're really consuming, and you may find yourself going nowhere fast.

Week 1 Steps to Success

1. Record your beginning weight, body composition measurements (if you're having a professional monitor your body fat percentage), and the suggested nutrient intake totals appropriate for you.

2. Plan a sample day by creating meals that include quality foods, meal volumes that are appropriate, and meal times that fit into your schedule. Adjust the meal amounts until the total amount of protein, carbohydrates, and fat fall into your suggested ranges at the end of the day.

3. Plan ahead for the day and make sure you have the food available that you'll need.

4. Record food intake throughout the day.

5. Make adjustments for the next day if necessary. This is the first week, so don't expect perfection.

6. At the end of the week weigh yourself. (Keep in mind that weight loss more than one to two pounds is water loss in the first week.)

7. Review your week and focus on lessons learned so you can improve next week.

8. Keep your Diet Docs' Rx card with you for quick reference.

Week 2

Now you have a great base of experience to know what all those grams of protein, carbohydrates, and fat really mean in a day of food intake. Week 2's objective is to refine your meals and work on making sure your program is going to be perfect for you. Chapter 6 offered guidance in creating meals that would be fairly consistent in volume, timing, and quality so that your body can best process the food you consume throughout the day. Blood chemistry stability is a major factor in how you'll feel and how effective your weight loss will be. You want to experience more energy than you thought possible and minimize your hunger. This is easily accomplished by focusing on the "nuts and bolts" of your food throughout the day.

This week will be a fair assessment of the amount of food you're consuming. The first week's weight loss was a combination of water loss and fat loss, but this week will allow a better look at actual *fat* loss. Two to three pounds for men and one to two pounds for women is about perfect. Faster loss may indicate that you're in danger of losing muscle, getting too hungry, and being prone to overeating. Review chapter 5 on how to adjust your nutrient numbers if you're losing too fast or too slowly.

Glance back through week 1's journal of your food intake. Check for the consistency of your daily numbers, spacing between meals, and meal volume. Are you too high or too low on protein, carbs, or fat? Were there some large gaps between meals (four hours or more)? As noted previously, we disagree with nutritionists who try to get people to have the exact same ratios and amounts of food at exact time intervals, but there does need to be some consistency. The amount of flexibility appropriate is based on your hunger patterns and schedule. (Scheduling issues are when you can eat a whole-food meal and when you may need a protein bar or shake.) These are elements for you to decide based on your social situation and based on your hunger, likes, and dislikes.

If you aren't seeing the results you want, you may have to revisit this step and make sure you're not sabotaging your progress out of convenience. Some foods may need to be sacrificed for you to progress.

Week 2 Steps to Success

1. Review your first week of journaling. Look at daily nutrient totals, meal spacing, and recall when you were hungry, your energy levels, and ease of meal consumption.

2. Alter your meal plans if necessary due to schedule inconvenience or hunger patterns. Experiment to improve your comfort level.

3. Purposely increase your variety of foods to expand your arsenal of potential meals and snacks.

4. Start journaling about how the diet is affecting you so you can relate your body's responses to what you're consuming.

5. Weigh yourself and determine if you're losing too fast or too slow. Adjust your program according to the information in chapter 5.

Week 3

Now you're over the hump and on your way to permanent success! Whether you realize it or not, you have altered your eating habits and have gained a great deal of valuable knowledge. Those first two weeks constitute the largest "structural" steps in your program. You have fine-tuned your food volume for a typical day that will satisfy proper nutritional needs to lose body fat and maintain lean body mass. If you're losing too fast or too slow, keep adjusting your totals based on the information in chapter 5. Excellent documentation of your nutrition is a key to making sure you have as objective a guide as possible.

Now it's time to look at the details of the food you're consuming. This is a good time to review chapter 2 and increase your understanding of carbohydrates. The amount of information can be a little overwhelming, but success in this area will come from the details. When you're dieting, the glycemic index, carbohydrate volume per meal, and avoiding sugar and trigger foods become paramount. You want small, rolling insulin fluctuations in your bloodstream not mountainous spikes. The closer you stick to the physiological principles, the easier it will be for you to succeed.

Carbohydrates are the body's primary energy source. At this point in your program, you may feel some hunger return if you're generally not eating enough calories. Most people believe they are eating more food than normal because of the increase in protein and fibrous carbohydrates and because "power spacing" helps them feel full (see chapter 6). However, it's also a common pattern for people to start letting protein levels slide and start increasing carbohydrate intake again. If you're heading in this direction, it's a slow path to a plateau. Keep your carbs in check because too much carbohydrate intake will block your body's need to use an alternative energy source—body fat.

Blood chemistry stability is a great focus. Make sure you're not elevating carbohydrates too high at meals or leaving gaping holes in your day without enough fuel. Look at your food journaling and make sure you have some balance in your meals and snacks. They don't have to be exact replicas of each other, but you should avoid major inconsistencies as you stay within your carbohydrate range for the day. Too many carbs in one meal and you'll be lethargic and then very hungry. Too few for too many hours and you'll also end up hungry and unable to pull in the reins at the kitchen table.

Week 3 Steps to Success

1. Review chapter 2 regarding carbohydrates.

2. Review your daily nutrition intake and take steps to make sure it's consistent.

3. Use a good measure of balance in your carbohydrate intake meal to meal. Avoid too many carbs in meals and don't allow too much time between meals so you're tempted to snack on whatever's convenient.

4. Start paying close attention to the glycemic index and note which carb sources trigger hunger a short while after the meal and which ones delay hunger.

5. Weigh yourself and adjust your nutrient intake as described in chapter 5 if necessary.

Week 4

Fat is a variable, second only to carbohydrates, that can be used to sustain body-fat loss if manipulated correctly. Chapter 3 provides plenty of detail regarding the function of fat in the body and the differences between "good" and "bad" fat.

Once you've created some good habits, including the addition of some healthy unsaturated fats, you'll need to cut the saturated fats to a minimum to stay within your daily range. If fat intake is as moderate as we suggest and healthy fats are the dominant source, then dietary fat will never earn the blame for lack of progress.

However, if the table starts tilting toward an increased fats intake (especially with a higher inclusion of saturated fats), a cascade of events will take place. First, the calorie-rich fat may take you right up to a maintenance range of food intake from your planned calorie deficit. This is common in people who mistakenly think carbs are the only thing to worry about. A hefty handful of almonds may seem like the best thing to eat to avoid letting the carbs get too high, but if the extra fat increases the total calories for the day beyond deficit range, a day of weight loss is missed. Portion size and daily food volume are critical steps.

Second, fat can be absorbed straight from the bloodstream and into your fat cells. Too much fat in a meal on a day in which calories weren't low enough results in a lack of progress and may lead to regaining a small amount of fat. Excessive amounts of fat can only be used as energy successfully if carbs are near zero, such as in a ketogenic diet. As previously discussed, this isn't the best or easiest way to lose weight. Make sure you're not letting your dietary fat grams climb by mistakenly focusing on carbs.

The bottom line is to make sure you include a variety of healthy unsaturated fats wherever you can in your diet. Keep fat sources spaced evenly throughout the day. Spacing will make it easier to stay in your suggested totals, allowing for slower digestion and better maintenance of blood glucose levels. More importantly, it helps keep hunger in check.

Week 4 Steps to Success

1. Pick a variety of unsaturated fats that can be used as at least 50 percent of your fat intake.

2. Space out fat intake as evenly as possible within your meal structure.

3. Don't let fat intake creep up just to keep carbs down.

4. Perform your weekly review of nutrition journaling for consistency, and check your weight for progress. Make your best effort to correct problem areas in carrying out your program and adjust your program if necessary (see chapter 5).

Week 5

Minimizing protein's role in weight loss is a mistake. As a matter of fact, behaviorally it's one of the best indicators of a client's success. Most people who embark on this journey will have to raise their protein to a level they're not used to. We certainly don't advocate an unsafe, unhealthy, or even unnecessary level of protein intake, but most of us just don't eat enough. That's a controversial statement since people can survive on very little, but we're after *thriving*, not surviving. Basal metabolic function requires approximately 50 to 70 grams of protein a day just to stay in "neutral," and that doesn't account for the potential increased needs due to the calorie deficit of dieting and exercise. So eat your protein!

When protein is consumed, it is digested slowly. Therefore other foods eaten at the same time are also digested and absorbed slowly. After those meals, blood chemistry will be more stable for a longer period. Hunger will be lower and energy will be higher. You don't have to eat protein at every meal, but there are some key times when protein is called for.

Breakfast, for instance, is a good time to eat some protein to prevent hunger shortly thereafter. If you can't eat much protein at breakfast, make sure you get some in your first snack, such as a protein bar or shake. Dinner is also a good meal to include a whole-food protein source to help prevent late-evening hunger. These two suggestions are based on years of experience as to what will help you succeed, but you should also be guided by your personal observations of your hunger patterns and schedule preferences.

It may have taken you a week or two to get your protein levels up to your suggested ranges. While weight loss is steady and energy is increasing, it is easy to ride this high because of the positive reinforcement. But eventually the rigors of daily life start competing with that momentum, and it's easier to make choices due to convenience instead of conviction. Protein intake starts decreasing, hunger increases, and carbohydrate consumption increases again. This is the recipe for slipping out of body fat burning mode.

Joe works with a lot of professional bodybuilders, and he will tell you that what works for them will work for you. When fat has to come off, eating enough protein absolves hunger, creates a more fat-loss-friendly internal environment, and pulls a lot of other functions into place.

You'll lose weight faster when you include a protein shake or two as snacks. Shakes or other protein-rich sources keep blood sugar stable, cut cravings, and save more fat and carbs for meals. You can eat a whole-food protein source as a snack as well. When you find it difficult to get enough protein, remember to choose habits that are easy to maintain.

Week 5 Steps to Success

1. Make sure your protein levels aren't sliding downward.

2. Keep protein sources lean whenever possible. Save fattier selections for occasional meals.

3. Consider protein bars or shakes for snacks if protein levels are difficult to achieve.

4. Review your charting and look for a link between lower-protein days and increased hunger and possible increases in carb intake.

5. Hunger often is preceded by low-protein meals. Consider increasing protein.

6. Check body weight for progress and adjust nutrient numbers per chapter 5 if necessary.

Week 6

You're now coasting through the middle portion of your weight-loss program! Reviewing all the key points in this six-week program from time to time will help keep the driving principles in the forefront of your mind. You may also consider reading certain chapters again for additional assessments of your progress.

Week 6 is dedicated to an evaluation of your progress and setting up a management plan for the rest of your time in weight-loss mode, which may be another 3, 6, or 18 months. After that you'll arrive at the incredible day of being able to celebrate the success of reaching your goal and increasing your food to maintenance levels.

To get there, keep your hands on the plow. Look at your daily charting of protein, carbohydrate, and fat intake. Carefully compare that information to your weight-loss progress. Pay attention to overall calorie intake. Calculate weekly averages for those statistics and look for the relationship between the level of food and macronutrients you're eating and your rate of weight loss. You should be able to see a causal relationship between the two. You can observe with clarity and precision how much food you can eat each day (on average) and lose one pound, two pounds, or whatever your healthy desired rate. This is one reason documentation is key to success. You have created a database that will enable you to manage your weight control for as long as you wish.

That is the goal for the remainder of your program. Decide what pace you want to continue on (based on recommendations of safe weight loss and your comfort level), and plan meals and daily nutritional totals accordingly.

Keep monitoring your progress and recording your food intake as you add to your knowledge. Understand that there will be an occasional setback or a social situation at which you anticipate not "eating perfectly" according to your plan, but if these are infrequent, your progress will continue.

Week 6 Steps to Success

1. Review weekly weight-loss rate and compare with weekly averages of all three macronutrients.

2. Compare the relationship of this data for accurate estimations of the food intake required for different rates of weekly weight loss.

3. Celebrate the completion of your first six weeks! (Yahooooooo!)

You're on Your Way

There you have it. Your prescription for the next six weeks…and the rest of your very healthy life. Prepare for a long-but-satisfying journey of experimentation, changes, new understanding, and better integration of proper nutrition into your daily life.

It's incredibly rewarding to see a client lose 34 or 35 pounds or to have a client reach the goal of losing 15 pounds in 8 weeks.

We are even more ecstatic when we see that client enjoying a higher quality of life a year later without having gained any weight back. This long-term success has very little to do with us. We take great pleasure in knowing that clients took the right information and worked consistently hard to win what were perhaps great wars in their lives. We can educate and motivate, but ultimately it's you who will or will not succeed. You may fall down once in a while, but you can get back up.

As the initial motivation wears off and the ice cream is no longer as easy to pass up, you have to remember who you're doing this for. You now have the tools to stick to the program. You have a plan that's a proven success. You're no longer stumbling around in the dark.

We know you can do it!

The Diet Docs in Action...

Mary's Story

Weighing myself is an exciting experience, and I love going to stores to find new jeans or bathing suits. All this is a dream come true for me, a person with a lifelong track record of disordered eating and dieting. Today I look and feel better at 40 than I ever have in my life. That's how it is with The Diet Docs.

On my own, I was fighting a losing battle. I'm not immune to the psychologically charged nature of food and eating in this culture. We celebrate our victories and soothe our losses with food. The pressure on women and girls to be "small and skinny" makes that struggle even harder. I am a large-framed woman—5'10" and wear a size 11 shoe. So small and skinny is not in the cards for me. However, since high school I made sad attempts to control my size that resulted in extreme disordered eating. My life revolved around dieting and the numbers on the scale. I hated my body. I tried every quick fix and popular diet you can think of. I would commence each program thinking, *This is the one,* only to gain fat. These popular diets also exaggerated the psychopathology behind my negative body image and disordered eating. My weight fluctuated, as did my dress size. I had no balance in my life, and this negatively impacted upon important relationships. My unhealthy dealings with food were exercises in futility.

After working closely with Dr. Joe I've learned I can be slender, athletic, and lean. The program gives me the proper tools to do this. There is no guesswork. My metabolism is ramped up, my lean body mass is stable, and my fat-burning capacity is at full speed. As a result, disordered eating has vanished, and I have carved out the body of a professional athlete. One of the greatest benefits is that I have maintained this for years now. I've even learned to handle events that arise, such as holidays, reunions, and other emotionally charged occasions.

Most important, I finally have a healthy relationship with food and balance around eating. I can be present and "in the moment" with my daughter and husband, and not always worried about weight. I am finally enjoying my life, my family, and taking pride in my body!

continued ➡

Never did I think that I would be a competitive athlete after 40, but I am! Never did I dream of having balance in my life with food, but I do! The notion of eating normally without fear, disorder, and fat gain was a dream. It's come true! Thank you, Dr. Joe, for your continued support, guidance, and believing in me. I owe my success to you!

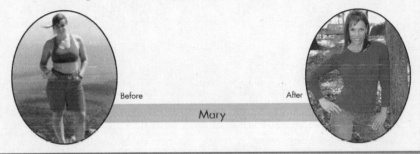

Before   After

Mary

CHAPTER 10

Great Health Benefits!

By now you've probably picked up the idea that this program is not *just* about losing weight but also about being healthy. And it just so happens that a trim body is more likely than an overweight body to be healthy. While it's true you can be fat and happy, you can't be fat and *healthy*.

If overweight people will commit to a *moderate* weight-loss program, it can improve their health. With that in mind, let's talk about some of the health consequences of poor diet and finish with how weight loss and proper nutrition can combat these.

The growing field of nutritional genomics is focusing on the key nutrients in food that affect us on a genetic level. Researchers hope to isolate these compounds to decrease disease risk, including coronary artery disease, cancer, and Alzheimer's. Let's look at some of the latest research from this field as we discuss how food can make us healthier.

Obesity

Obesity is truly an epidemic in this country. Evidence is now showing that it may eventually replace smoking as the number one cause of preventable death in the United States. Seemingly every study starts with a "gloom and doom" paragraph about the direction our country is heading in regard to expanding our waistlines. Here's a sample platter of these statistics:

- More than 60% of U.S. adults are overweight or obese (having a Body Mass Index, or BMI, greater than 25 for women and 30 for men).

- The prevalence of adult obesity increased an unbelievable 57% between 1991 and 1999.

- The prevalence of adult (type II) diabetes climbed 765% from 1935 to 1996.

- 47 million Americans may have metabolic syndrome in addition to the problems of heart disease, stroke, and arthritis.

The statistics are so grim at times people are tempted to put their heads in the sand and believe the lie that they can't do anything about these problems. But we can and we must take action. The numbers reveal this is a war we need to win so future generations won't be burdened with unimaginable health-care costs.

The nature of obesity is that it is a chronic, relapsing illness that is never cured. We can stop smoking and drinking, but we can't stop eating. We must decide to make sure what is going into our systems is good for us. Obesity *is* controllable.

An Agent of Change

Food is the "agent" that acts on the "host" (that would be you and me) to produce disease. Ideally we would like to use food to *prevent* or *cure* diseases rather than it being an agent that causes it.

Scientists are discovering that the substances in food not only affect us now, but act upon our genes (nutritional genomics). Within the next 10 years it may be possible to genetically map individuals who may be at risk for certain illnesses. (Sounds exciting but would you want to know if you were at a higher risk for cancer or Alzheimer's? Would it change the way you live? Even more important, would you want your insurance company to know? What about the person who knows and yet chooses to live an unhealthy lifestyle? An interesting bioethics debate, don't you think?)

Since we don't have a crystal ball, we'll talk about some of the known illnesses and how certain foods and weight loss may affect them. One hopeful article appeared in the January 17, 2005 issue of *Newsweek*. One of the top researchers in genetics was discussing a particular gene variant (Apo E4) that increases the risk of diabetes, coronary artery disease (CAD), and Alzheimer's. The article stated that "15 to 30% of the population may contain at least one copy of this allele...but if you stop smoking, give up alcohol, exercise, and eat a diet low in saturated fat you can remove *all* genetic predisposition for heart disease that comes with E4." Not just some, but *all* of it. Food is powerful medicine, but its administration has to be tempered with the realities of everyday living, which is why we are giving you structure with flexibility rather than an exact, precise regimen for every single meal and snack for every single second of every single day.

The following discussion cannot be an all-inclusive list or expect to provide the detailed information of hundreds of pages of studies and entire chapters from medical textbooks; however, we hope it will highlight the important aspects of how nutrition and exercise can affect health.

Osteoarthritis, Fibromyalgia, and Chronic Fatigue Syndrome

Osteoarthritis is a very complicated problem, and we still don't have definitive answers for all the causes of premature breakdown of joint cartilage. Some people who have been quite thin their whole lives have arthritis and some extremely heavy people don't seem to have any problems with their joints. Exercise and nutrition do play a role in slowing the disease process. How obesity affects the joints may be a simple lesson in physics: more weight on the joint results in it breaking down faster. Muscles help reduce stress on cartilage, so keeping the muscles strong and the joints mobile further help to reduce pain and degeneration. Not getting enough calcium, vitamin D, and magnesium may further harm joints as well as accelerate other physical problems. Where do we get these magic nutrients? Lean dairy, fish, and produce. Glucosamine, a popular supplement, is basically a protein that helps to strengthen and lubricate joints. (To learn how this supplement became so popular, read Jason Theodosakis' *The Arthritis Cure*.)

A brief aside about vitamin D: Top researchers in the field are becoming distressed at the decrease in the proper production of natural vitamin D (which is produced when our skin is exposed to sunlight) as we spend more time indoors or slather on sunscreen. Dietary vitamin D has declined as we shun dairy and orange juice in our quest for lower carbs. Vitamin D has been shown to have positive affects on breast, prostate, and ovarian cancer, as well as rheumatoid arthritis, osteoporosis, and multiple sclerosis. Multiple sclerosis (MS) has long been known to occur more frequently in the northern latitudes, and one of the postulates is that MS is due to decreased sun and the consequent decrease in vitamin D production. Obviously the disease is more complicated than this, but it brings up interesting ideas.

One of the most fit individuals whom Scott worked with in medical residency was almost 15 years older than the other residents, but every day at lunch, in addition to his fish and veggies, he always had two cartons of skim milk. He could run circles around his younger collegues. Calcium has been shown to promote weight loss and has long been known to build strong bones and teeth and give you a shiny coat. That's why so many doctors play golf—it's for the vitamin D, baby!

Moderate physical exercise is also helpful to maintain joint mobility. If you're leaner and your muscles are stronger, your joints will hurt less. Orthopedic surgeons often will not perform joint replacements, especially total knee replacements, if a patient is substantially overweight. They know that the increased weight will decrease the longevity of the joint and significantly increase the post-operative complication rates. One of the coolest things I saw while on this program were local surgeons often referring people to Joe to help them lose weight before their operations so they would have the highest level of success. One such patient received a new knee after losing 50 pounds and then went on to have his other knee replaced after a second 50-pound drop. His surgeon is thrilled to see him riding his mountain bike in his sixth decade of life after many years of being sedentary and pain-ridden.

Exercise, along with physical therapy, has clearly been shown to improve fibromyalgia and chronic fatigue syndrome. Fibromyalgia syndrome (FMS) frequently occurs concurrently with arthritis. Often the strain on the muscle that protects the irritated joint will get sore. Proper nutrition helps the muscle, along with exercise and treatment such as physical therapy, massage, or chiropractic. These activities also can help decrease chronic muscle pain without having to take a bunch of pills. Many nonweight bearing or low-impact exercises are now available for people who can't do regular walking, jogging, and aerobics. Water aerobics, spinning classes, and recumbent exercise bikes, along with the favorite elliptical trainer, are available in almost any gym and are becoming more affordable. Certain insurance companies will, at times, pay for exercise classes, rehabilitation classes, or physical therapy for people with certain diagnoses such as osteoarthritis or cardiac disease. (Check with your physician before starting an exercise program!) These classes provide an excellent supervised way to get started. Joe recalls a client with the diagnosis of FMS who had a history of three whiplash-type injuries. Two minutes on a stationary bike landed her in bed for a week after their first meeting. Light massage therapy, pain meds, and every treatment imaginable were a way of life for her. It took a slow, arduous year of progressive therapeutic exercise combined with a thorough overhaul of her nutrition, but this client ended up returning to work without pain. She now enjoys vigorous workouts!

Chronic fatigue syndrome is poorly understood and has created unbelievable debate in the medical community as to its causes and treatment. B vitamins can certainly help and are found in whole grains, vegetables, and supplements. Viruses have also been postulated to play a role, and some factions have wanted the illness renamed "CFIDS" for "chronic fatigue immune deficiency syndrome." (We won't get into that debate.) Eating right and exercising will improve fatigue and your ability to fight diseases. First, decreasing the excessive amount of carbs in your diet will decrease your insulin spikes that make you tired after eating a meal. Second, keeping the sugar level in your bloodstream down allows your immune cells to work better. This is one of the reasons why diabetics have trouble fighting disease. The excessive sugar in their bloodstream slows proper migration and function of their white blood cells. Although you may not be diabetic, by eating too many carbs and calories, your body's constant clearing of so much sugar will impair your disease-fighting ability. This is part of the reason why people who are overweight and eat poorly seem to have more colds than their skinny-mini, Bowflex-hugging friends.

High Cholesterol, Cardiovascular Disease, and Hypertension

Cholesterol and You

The result of consuming lipids (fats) seems pretty straightforward. If you eat too many, the excess gets stuffed into your fat cells, or even worse, they get stuck in your arteries. Pretty basic. True, there is a segment of the population whose lipids may eventually decrease after severely limiting carbs and eating mainly protein and fat instead. However, we have already established how difficult it is to maintain this type of diet for any clinically relevant length of time. For some people, low-carb dieting will result in their lipids increasing. It's very difficult when you don't know how your body will react, and this isn't a small gamble! The huge majority of evidence confirms that excessive fat in our diet is not good for us.

We should not advocate a high-carb diet, but neither should we advocate a diet high in animal fat and cholesterol. Besides increasing our blood lipids, a diet high in animal fat—especially heavily grilled meats—may increase our risk of certain types of cancer, such as colorectal. It is critically important to know your entire lipid panel (not just your total cholesterol) because a decent total cholesterol may give a false sense of security. Scott once had a physician friend who had his first heart attack when his cholesterol was 150, well below the recommended 200. However, his "good" cholesterol was only 15 at the time.

Cholesterol panels are broken down into the following: Total Cholesterol (TC), Triglycerides, High-Density Lipoproteins (HDL—the "good" or protective cholesterol), and Low-Density Lipoprotein (LDL—the arch villains of the cholesterol world).

It is important to know your entire panel because a poor LDL/HDL ratio can indicate higher risk. Decreasing fat in your diet can help reduce LDL and TC. Decreasing carbs can help lower triglycerides. Finally, exercise can help raise HDL (one of the few things that can raise HDL short of medication) and positively influence the rest of the cholesterol panel.

Some vitamins (such as niacin) can decrease triglycerides and raise HDL. "Statin drugs," or HMG Co-A reductase inhibitors (say that three times fast!), are the primary drugs used to lower LDL. They go by many popular names: Lipitor, Pravachol, Zocor, and Crestor, to name a few.

If you can't get your lipids under control on our diet program, it's probably indicative that you have genetic factors influencing your blood chemistry. Thankfully there are compounds that can prolong your life. Create your own metabolic transformation by faithfully following this program and exercising, and we believe most of you can avoid the medicine chest. But don't be afraid of medication if you need it. Combined with exercise and good nutrition, you'll be using the least amount possible.

Cardiovascular Issues

Newer markers such as very low-density lipoprotein (VLDL), homocysteine levels, and highly selective, or cardiac C-reactive protein (c-CRP), are being studied as potential detectors for coronary disease. The most important may eventually turn out to be c-CRP because it is a marker for inflammation. Inflammation seems to accelerate the laying down of athrogenic plaques (that gooey stuff inside your arteries that causes them to narrow and increases your risk for a heart attack) and several illnesses, including Alzheimer's disease, MS, and autoimmune disease. Diet and exercise can positively impact the lipids as well as inflammation. Increasing your blood circulation with exercise helps to pull oxygen and nutrients to all parts of your body so that free radicals and pro-inflammatory substances find it much harder to maintain a foothold.

Hypertension

Hypertension (high blood pressure) can be significantly impacted by weight status. If you carry lots of extra adipose (you don't have to cart it out in a little red wagon like Oprah did, but you get the picture), your body has to make plenty of extra blood vessels to help keep that fatty tissue alive. Your heart has to pump that much harder to force blood through those miles of extra vessels, and your blood pressure goes up (somewhat of a simplistic explanation, but that's what it boils down to). Shrink the fat, and you decrease the strain on your pump.

Furthermore, if you're eating a healthy diet, you won't be eating a lot of processed food or foods with a lot of extra salt. Salt may not have a lot of bearing on certain people with hypertension, but there is a percentage of the population with hypertension, edema (swelling), and congestive heart failure who experience increased blood pressure with higher sodium intake. If you have high blood pressure, take it easy on the salt. People often mistakenly think that since they aren't using the salt shaker they aren't getting much salt in their diet. Read labels and pay attention to sodium content if you have these types of problems. Certain soups, processed foods, and snacks have significant levels of sodium. People wind up in the hospital with a flare-up of their congestive heart failure if they are careless with their sodium consumption. They eat pretzels knowing they are low-fat and pat themselves on the back about avoiding the high-fat chips (which is good), but they don't realize how much sodium they're putting away with their Mister Saltys.

Remember, you are on your way to becoming your own nutritionist. Good health involves knowing proteins, carbs, and fats and also sodium, potassium, and caffeine content if you are at risk. Reducing hypertension through proper diet and exercise helps decrease the acceleration of atherosclerosis of the arteries and ultimately coronary disease. Now you know why your doctor is always on you to keep your weight and blood pressure down. All of those things go hand in hand to slow the buildup of plaque in the arteries.

In addition to eating less fat and cholesterol and increasing exercise, certain foods—including fish oil, walnuts, flaxseed oil, and good ol' broccoli—will help decrease lipids and cardiovascular risk. To return to our discussion of nutritional genomics, broccoli has been shown to influence the gene GST, which helps produce the body's main antioxidant, glutathione. This decreases cancer risk and helps keep arteries healthy. Antioxidants help fight free radicals produced in the body that may lead to inflammation or certain types of cancers. And as we've already discussed, no one wants inflamed (or even somewhat incensed or indignant) arteries in his or her body.

Cancer

Nothing strikes fear in the heart like the word "cancer." This is such a loaded and complicated subject that we considered not including it. However, we do think we need to make some judicious comments.

We don't want anyone to think that if people with cancer are overweight they "gave" themselves the disease or that it is their fault. This malady is far too complex to give such a glib answer. Also, thin people, including world-class athletes, get cancer too. Look at the wonderful triumph of Lance Armstrong. (One of the drugs that helped cure him came from tree bark.)

Furthermore, we would not want people to abandon proven scientific treatment to rely only on nutrition for a cure. However, several links between obesity and cancer have been drawn and confirmed. Increased weight can help certain tumors survive and grow. Good nutrition can positively affect your treatment, whereas poor nutrition can increase risk factors.

One recent study showed that eating french fries just twice a week increased the risk of breast cancer 27 times. Soybeans affect 123 genes involved in prostate cancer and help block tumor formation. And we've already talked about broccoli and vitamin D.

As our friends in research continue to pound away, stay tuned on how the food you put into your body every day can help decrease your risk of cancer. There are already volumes of comprehensive books detailing the micronutritional content of certain foods and their positive effects on cancer prevention and their curative properties. Guess what foods make up, oh, about 99.9 percent of this list? Fruits and vegetables.

Diabetes Type II

Diabetes mellitus type II (DM II) and metabolic syndrome are two diseases significantly affected by weight. Approximately 90 percent of diabetes is noninsulin dependent, otherwise known as diabetes type II, or adult onset diabetes.

Genetics obviously influence our ability to get these diseases, and the good news, according to textbooks and recent studies, is that even moderate weight loss (as little as 10 pounds) may significantly decrease the risk of the disease and also limit its impact on your health.

As we discussed earlier, exercise will decrease cardiovascular risk, assist in losing body fat, and reduce your BMI (body mass index), and it will also decrease your diabetes risk. Exercise will also positively influence DM II, but not as much as if incorporated with weight loss.

The epidemiology of DM II makes it critical that we continue to work to defeat this disease. Our rapidly increasing waistlines result in an increase in DM II cases. Conservative studies show that DM II accounts for about 15 percent of health care costs in the United States, and its consequences can be tragically debilitating.

According to the *Cecil Textbook of Medicine*, "[DM II] is the leading cause of blindness, end-stage renal disease, and nontraumatic limb amputations." Furthermore, it increases cardiovascular complications, peripheral vascular disease, and neuropathy, a very painful, chronic burning condition in the extremities. The scary thing is that the symptoms for DM II such as excessive thirst, excessive urination, weight loss, blurred vision, and dizziness may be subtle and missed or ignored for a long time. Some texts and studies speculate there may be an undiagnosed diabetic for every known case.

This is one disease you need to be tested for regularly if you are overweight, especially if you carry fat around your middle or if there is a family history of the disease. Even better, keeping your weight down throughout your life will significantly reduce your risk.

Diabetes is a combination of decreased insulin secretion and increased insulin resistance. Insulin resistance is clearly linked to obesity. In other words, a life of eating too many carbohydrates, which causes too much insulin to be secreted, and carrying too much weight will cause your whole body to become desensitized.

Diet and weight loss combined is truly the key to DM II avoidance and management. Treating diabetes is like a triangle: the three parts of the triangle are diet, physical activity, and medication. If you neglect any part of that triangle, the other two parts have to be stretched to make up for that deficiency. Diet and activity are within your control! Even if you have to start taking medicine, diet and exercise should be paramount. Keeping fat and carbs lower and lean protein higher is important. Weight reduction will help keep your blood glucose in check. Exercise will cause your body to use blood sugar as energy, thus keeping overall blood sugar lower. Even though you can't eliminate DM II (yet!), keeping these two parts of the triangle under control may delay the need for medication or result in a decreased dose.

In disease states such as hypertension, diabetes, and hyperlipidemia, you must keep your sugar, lipids, and blood pressure under the tightest control for the longest time possible. Most of the damage caused by these illnesses is cumulative over time. Though you may be able to eliminate or avoid a lot of medication, which is your goal, you need to take medicine if your doctor prescribes it and use it until he or she says otherwise. There is no sense having a disease, going to your doctor, and then just halfway controlling it. Your doctor will welcome your active participation in increasing the quality and length of your life. Work with your physician if you want to have the greatest, healthiest life span possible.

Alzheimer's

The physiology of Alzheimer's is still not completely understood, and older Americans are rightly fearful of the words "Alzheimer's disease." What do we know? Curry powder contains turmeric, which has been shown to suppress genes that increase inflammation. Inflammation has been implicated in heart disease and colon cancer and Alzheimer's. India has one of the lowest incidences of Alzheimer's in the world, and the use of turmeric for seasoning is thought to play a role in that low occurrence. Exercise and anti-inflammatories may also positively affect this disease. Mental activity, such as reading and doing crossword puzzles, stimulates your brain and can slow even normal neurological aging. Physical exercise increases the blood flow that carries healthy nutrition directly to the brain. As we've already stressed, a diet low in sugar and fat causes less inflammation than does a diet high in sugar and fat. It's more complicated than this, but there is cause for optimism.

The Granddaddy of Them All: Metabolic Syndrome

What is "metabolic syndrome," and why should we care? Metabolic syndrome is one of the fastest growing diseases in the United States. The illness has gone by a number of names in the past, including syndrome X, dysmetabolic syndrome, and insulin resistance syndrome. This condition entails abdominal obesity, abnormal lipids, elevated blood pressure, insulin resistance, a prothrombotic state (making you more prone to blood clots), and a pro-inflammatory state (remember how serious inflammation can be).

If you get metabolic syndrome, you will be on the fast track to heart disease and diabetes. How fast, you ask? Scott has seen patients with metabolic syndrome as young as their late 30s and early 40s with full-blown heart disease that required intervention such as angioplasty or open heart surgery. A recent study from the *Third National Health and Nutrition Examination Survey* stated that 47 million Americans have metabolic syndrome. Good grief, Charlie Brown! That's 24 percent of the U.S. population! Have you ever seen the bill for a cardiac catheter? On an even more serious note, one in four heart attacks result in death. That's right folks, death. No guys with paddles, no family members patting your hand in the ICU. Dead, gone. It's not well-publicized, but that's a fact, Jack.

So how is this disease state defined? For men, an abdominal waist circumference greater than 40 inches and for women, greater than 35 inches starts your membership in this dubious club. (Run get that tape measure! And this doesn't mean the smallest pair of jeans you can squeeze yourself into before you pass out from asphyxia.) Further criteria include triglycerides > 150; HDL < 40 for men and < 50 for women; blood pressure > 130/85, and finally, fasting glucose > 110. People who have any three of the five criteria qualify as having metabolic syndrome. Obesity, lack of activity, and genetic factors all contribute to the illness, and excessive body fat and inactivity accelerate the expression of those genes.

We can't trade our genes in for a new set just yet. As stated in an article in *Contemporary Management of Metabolic Syndrome,* "The greatest potential of benefit from management of metabolic syndrome lies in reversing its root causes: overweight/obesity and physical inactivity." Why is eliminating obesity important? "Abdominal/ visceral adiposity is associated with an increased release of free fatty acids into the portal blood, which, in turn, leads to hepatic over-production of triglycerides and decreased synthesis of high-density lipoprotein cholesterol, both characteristic of metabolic syndrome." In other words, having a fat tummy releases toxins in your system and decreases your body's ability to produce the good stuff to fight those toxins. (Now that sounds a little nicer than that complicated scientific jargon, doesn't it?)

The long and the short of it is that if we are carrying a lot of weight in our abdomen and chest, that fatty tissue is releasing substances that will harm us. This is why people with the "apple" shape rather than the "pear" shape need to get to their physicians and not just their plastic surgeons. Increased weight increases insulin resistance, which in turn will increase blood sugar, blood pressure, and negative lipid profiles. Since the receptors on the tissues are not as sensitive, your body has to pump out more and more insulin to get the same response. We've discussed how excessive insulin is an enemy, and this condition quickly turns into a vicious cycle of insulin resistance, increased insulin, weight gain, and then further insulin release!

This will eventually lead to DM II and all the problems that go along with that. Hypertension is at least twice as common in patients with DM II as it is in patients without the disease. Furthermore, patients with hypertension are twice as likely to develop diabetes over a four-to-five year period. Hypertension then accelerates the complications of diabetes, especially stroke, kidney disease, and diabetic eye disease.

So what can we do to stop the slide?

Um, how 'bout diet and exercise? And it doesn't matter what age you are. One 5,000-person study showed that intentional weight loss in people with metabolic syndrome decreased mortality by 25 percent.

Another study in the *American Journal of Preventative Medicine* showed that "104 adults aged 55 to 75 reduced their rate of metabolic syndrome by 41% after 6 months by adding 20 minutes of weightlifting to their aerobic routine." We see plenty of older people at the gym hitting the machines. They may not have abs like LL Cool J, and sometimes the big ol' bodybuilders get a little annoyed that granny is monopolizing their machine, but these folks are exercising!

Studies like these prove that older people can improve their health, so go drink a protein shake, sonny, and come back in a few minutes.

Dropping as few as 10 pounds and reducing blood pressure by 10 points can decrease the damage from these diseases. Indeed, some studies have gone so far as to indicate that if we achieve optimal control over the risk factors, the disease may be reduced by 80 percent. Food (and exercise) for thought.

Nutritional Genomics

Exciting developments are expected from nutritional genomics. Ever since Dr. Sears talked about "eicosanoids," the friendly little quarks of the nutritional world, a bridge between science and the lay person's understanding of nutrition has developed. This field holds the most promise as scientists isolate the chemicals in food and the particular genes they act on. This will help take a bit of the nebulous nature out of nutrition and pin down some hardcore pathways for benefiting our bodies.

The next vexing question, however, is, How much should we eat of certain things? Will a pound of broccoli a day be enough to cut down disease risks? And if that's what it takes, do you want to be the one who sits next to that broccoli-eating person on the bus?

Ending the Fitness Versus Fatness Debate

Two key articles were presented in the *Journal of the American Medical Association (JAMA)* at the end of 2004. To summarize, it appears that physical inactivity is the main risk factor for cardiovascular disease, and a high body mass index (BMI) is the main risk factor for diabetes. They each influence the other to a certain degree, but this is the direction these studies pointed to. This research was in women, so stand in line, guys. We can conjecture logically that there will probably be a correlation in men (how strong remains to be seen).

The guy in the Bowflex commercial is calling out Jared about eating Subway sandwiches. We love Jared, and he and Subway have raised nutrition awareness extensively in the fast-food sector. Food versus exercise doesn't have to be like the North and the South with the Yankees of diet and the Confederates of exercise. You need both. Don't think that if you haven't achieved six-pack abs yet that you are a failure either. We often run into people's rationalization, "Hey, I exercise. I can eat what I want" or "I eat healthy. I don't need to exercise." As we've discussed, you must have *both* for total health.

Health Doesn't Care

Now, let's be very, very clear about something. No one should be prejudiced against people who are overweight. All people deserve to be loved and respected. We shouldn't look down on overweight people. But we do need to acknowledge that being overweight even moderately will put us at higher risk for significant health problems. Study after study has shown that. We all know of the person who smoked too much, drank too much, or ate too much and lived to be 100. But we can tell you story after story of people who were substantially overweight and it cost them their lives in their 30s and 40s. And then there are all the days of using canes, walkers, wheel chairs, oxygen tanks, hospital beds, and the general debility that often accompany serious weight problems.

If you are not exercising and not putting proper fuel into your body, you are missing out on optimal health. We should love ourselves enough to take care of ourselves. You see, "health" doesn't care. Health doesn't care if your father or mother was mean or cruel to you growing up. Health doesn't care that you hate your job or that life is stressful. It doesn't care; it just is what it is.

You can love yourself fat or thin, and you can pretty much hate yourself fat or thin. Step out of denial at both extremes and get the help you need physically and emotionally. Love yourself enough to get healthy. Scott has known his wife since high school, which covers a 155- to 230-pound weight swing and all spaces in between. She has always loved him no matter what his weight. Love was never the issue. But as his blood pressure reached 170/105, she was gravely concerned about his health. Scott didn't love himself enough to care about the imminent risks to his well being. That is a big and common problem. Until he cared about the *reality* of his declining physical health, he wouldn't put much energy into caring for himself.

Now you say, "But guys, I may be 30, 40, or 50 pounds over-weight, but I don't smoke or drink and my blood pressure and lipids are good. I exercise three or four days a week. What's the problem?" The problem is the evidence from the studies we've cited. The evidence is unblinking and unflinching and comes with no malice or prejudice. You may be fine now, but you have significantly increased your risk of future problems. Scott sincerely believes that his years of poor eating habits, along with his excessive weight, has shortened his life span. He can do everything now in his power to reverse that trend, but there is some damage that has been done that can't be reversed. That doesn't mean he's not going to try or that he's going to say, "What the heck" and go with the flow. Scott wants to stick around for his wife and children and the people he cares for on a day-to-day basis. Dying versus living healthy—compare and contrast that for a while.

Key Points

1. Good nutrition is critical for good health. Duh.

2. Nutrition can affect you even at the genetic level. (Now that's heavy duty.)

3. Weight affects your diabetes risk. Exercise can affect your cardiovascular risk. And your knee bone connects to your thigh bone...

4. Remember: Health doesn't care, so you should.

The Diet Docs in Action...

Phyllis & Wayne's Story

The Diet Docs' program has greatly impacted our health as well as our life. Dr. Uloth recommended we consult Dr. Joe after I developed Type II Diabetes and my husband began to develop high cholesterol, high blood pressure, and was unable to do the activities he enjoyed doing. Upon beginning the program January 2007, Wayne's weight was 341.1 pounds and my weight was 193.3 pounds. With Dr. Joe's instruction, The Diet Docs' book, and keeping a daily journal of our protein, carbohydrates, and fats, we started losing weight. As we weighed ourselves every week at Dr. Uloth's office and lost weight, we felt better, looked better, and definitely had more energy. Friends and family started commenting on our transformation. We were able to walk longer distances and exercise more than we had in a long time. After 8 months on the program, we had a combined total weight *loss* of 146.9 pounds, with Wayne weighing 227.4 pounds and me weighing 160.1 pounds. Wayne went from a waist size 54 to a size 40, and a shirt size of 4XL to a regular XL. I've gone from a size 18 to a size 10. The exciting thing is that we aren't done yet!

continued ⟶

This program is not a diet. It is a nutritional and metabolic way to change your eating habits. By understanding what you're eating and by making better nutritional choices, the weight will come off. Dr. Joe and Dr. Uloth were always there to offer guidance, support, and encouragement. The Diet Docs' book was great to reinforce motivation. The book offered recipes and ideas for preparing healthy meals. Watching the weight come off and feeling the extra energy as well as the health benefits of this program are not to be denied. My glucose levels have reduced to an excellent level, and I have been able to reduce my medications. My cholesterol levels have improved, and we both have seen significant decrease in our blood pressure.

This is a plan anyone can incorporate into his or her lifestyle. With the knowledge given in this book, and by learning to make healthier choices, we are still able to go out to eat, attend cookouts, birthday parties, and socialize with friends. Thanks to Dr. Joe and Dr. Uloth, we can now look forward to a much healthier and active lifestyle. Thanks, Diet Docs!

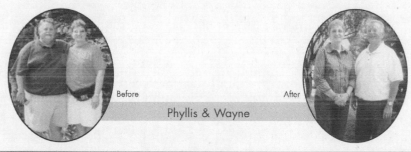

Before   After

Phyllis & Wayne

CHAPTER 11

Pitfalls and Obstacles

Sometimes when you're navigating a new diet plan you feel like you're swinging on vines over the gaping mouths of alligators below. Dieting has its pitfalls and obstacles. Let's take a look at some of the most common ones. These areas may seem quite obvious and others may be like quicksand. Even after you fall into one of these traps you may be left slapping your head and asking, *How could I have done that? How could I have been so stupid?*

Don't worry. We've all been here at one time or another. Your best defense against pitfalls is to make like a Scout and be prepared. You *will* face temptations, so plan ahead how you will handle them. Also keep yourself well-supplied with good foods that are easy to take with you.

Even better, arm yourself with the knowledge contained in these pages so you can make good choices no matter where you are. Do you remember the first Indiana Jones movie, *Raiders of the Lost Ark*? (You know, the good one; not the one where he is sitting around with the future Mrs. Spielberg eating monkey brains.) Picture that great fight scene in the market. We want you to be like Indiana Jones with a holster full of dietary knowledge and your diet foes to be like the big dude with the sword who didn't stand a chance. (And no, we don't know the protein count for monkey brains.)

"I don't have enough time to do all this!"

Being busy is a popular excuse. People tell us they are too busy when we discuss how they can eat healthier. It's always the same— poor eye contact, nodding heads in agreement, and a "But..." We know they're humoring us. If people have time to stop at a fast-food place or any type of grocery store, they aren't too busy, just making poor choices.

How about you? Is this your excuse? Well, even convenience stores have something healthy. At fast-food outlets you can order a chicken sandwich, side salad, and water or the burger, fries, and a large Coke. It's your choice. Your vocal cords can speak either sets of words. But are you more like Gollum in *The Lord of the Rings* saying, "Me wants it! Me needs it!" Think about your choices *before* you are faced with temptation. You can choose wisely.

Too many of us live as if we don't have a microsecond to spend on ourselves. We're busy people, after all. Yes, some of us *are* unbelievably busy, but we always seem to make time for what's important. Make time for this.

Check your cabinets and see how much healthy food you have right now. If you're well-stocked, simply allow a little more time at the store as you ponder a variety of healthy choices. If you don't have much at home, make a trip to the market now. Strike while the iron is hot! Take that enthusiasm you have for losing weight and use it to your advantage. Procrastination only leads to more excuses.

Also, remove any food from the house that may be a temptation. Periodically clean out any unhealthy foods that have accumulated from parties, restaurants, and the like. Some professionals advocate putting the kids' junk food in an out-of-the-way place to make it harder to get. We don't recommend that strategy for several reasons.

First of all, the first few weeks of the diet are crucial, so the kids and your spouse may just have to live a little sugar-deprived for that time. Second, you will hopefully be trying to get your kids to eat healthy as well. The only thing you are depriving them of is an early start on obesity, diabetes, and heart disease.

Finally, you *know* where the "junk drawer" is unless you've watched *50 First Dates* one too many times. Scott has been known to rappel from the ceiling like Tom Cruise in *Mission Impossible* to get that last Hershey Kiss his wife has hidden on the top shelf in the closet. Although it was fun trying to outsmart her, it was ultimately a game. If he wanted to be serious, he had to stop playing those kinds of games. Let's face it—he couldn't outwit her anyway. We know the junk is there; we also know we can grab anything we want at the gas station. Develop the discipline of avoidance.

Preparation really is crucial. True, it takes more time to clean a bunch of grapes than pop open a box of crackers or a bag of chips, but wash the grapes ahead of time and store them in the refrigerator. Then you can throw a few in your mouth when you're hungry. Nature's prepackaging of grapes, berries, and apples makes for a very quick snack. Fruit does have carbs, but any diet that makes you believe fruit isn't healthy is a joke. Too many carbs are bad for you, but the few carbs in a handful of blueberries are nothing in comparison to white bread or a potato. Also, fruit is high in antioxidants and fiber.

People who are health conscious often grill many chicken breasts ahead of time so they can quickly warm one in the microwave and have a meal or snack. You may not feel like cooking in advance, but it will help you save time later when you really need it.

Buy in bulk once you know what you like. We're not talking about buying the 50-gallon drum size you know will go bad after you only use a third of it. We're talking about buying two or three weeks of shakes, bars, frozen meals—whatever will be some of your mainstays—so you won't run out of ammunition.

You are developing a lifetime of eating and exercise habits, so don't expect to look like a cover model in a few weeks. That's completely unrealistic. Lasting results only come with time. Learn a little more each week. Many people believe that it takes anywhere from one to two months to really get "dialed in" on the nutritional and exercise points. After a few weeks you should feel very confident about what your body can do. The ensuing months will "toughen" you up as you settle in for the long haul. You will also see how you can enjoy certain foods without leading to a disaster...unless they are a "trigger food."

"All I had was one little scoop of ice cream and I was a goner!"

Is there anyone who *doesn't* have a trigger food? Trigger foods are edibles that if you start eating them, you have a terrible time stopping. To borrow a famous potato chip phrase, "Bet you can't eat just one." Don't mess with fire, and don't tempt fate. I've seen people with amazing willpower who can eat a few bites of cake or chocolate, but these people are few and far between.

Avoid trigger foods entirely, especially during the first several weeks of your diet. Even during your weekly "splurge meal" start practicing moderation. Later, as you enter maintenance, you will have learned to manage those foods without sabotaging yourself.

Trigger foods often are full of carbs that cause huge insulin spikes. If you succumb, you will then want to eat more and more, and you may find the cravings that had vanished during your months of healthy eating have returned with a vengeance. This reveals a fallacy of very low-carb diets—we are never really cured of our "carb addiction." Carbs release brain chemicals that make us feel good. We *want* them. The best we can hope for is to *control* our intake. If we let carbs get too low, our brains don't work well and we get grouchy. (Just ask Joe's wife when he's dieting for the Mr. International contest. Tracy has threatened to send him to live with us more than once during those times.) If we eat too few carbs over an extended period of time, important hormones get low, our metabolism falls, and we don't feel well. Make sure you eat the proper amount of carbs to avoid these pitfalls.

"It's not working anymore."

For some people, the greatest deterrent to achievement is reaching too high a comfort level too soon. Joe occasionally has clients who start with the incredible motivation that comes with the new understanding of nutrition and exercise. They start losing two to three pounds a week, refer friends to his practice, and are overjoyed with the results. These clients meticulously document food and nutrient totals and consistently do their exercises. And they make great progress toward their goal.

Then one day their progress slows. Sometimes they regain weight. All of a sudden "it's just not working anymore." They've probably just hit a plateau.

When you hit a plateau (and you will), first of all, don't give up. Second, problem solve. If you haven't lost enough, why is that? Have you not been documenting, watching your portion size, or reading your labels? Also, if you gained, it may not have been from what you ate the day before, but perhaps several days before, especially if it had high fat content. Sodium status may have affected your weight. (Did you pay a little visit to the Chinese buffet or the chip basket at the Mexican restaurant?)

When Joe asks to see their journals, the reply is often, "Well, I quit writing things down last month." Translation: "I've lost my motivation. I'm cheating. I'm no longer doing what needs to be done."

As soon as they get back on track, guess what? Their results pick right up where they left off. The point is that you must be consistent to reach your goal. It's so easy to slip upward into "maintenance" eating too soon. You're still eating the right percentages of macronutrients, but you're adding just a little too much food and the intake volume may take you out of the losing range and into the maintenance range prematurely.

Stick with your weight-loss level of food intake for as long as you can and then take a planned break. That's when you increase your volume to a maintenance level to "catch your breath," regroup, and then go right back to progressing. Your initial progress needs to be underscored by *consistency*.

So many variables affect your weight. Don't give up! If you're losing one to two pounds a week, you're doing great! You may lose at a much faster clip initially, but most people eventually settle into a healthy and sustainable one to two pounds per week pace. That is a perfect rate to keep weight off permanently.

Isn't it easier to stay at 140 now instead of hovering at 150? You bet it is. Don't weigh yourself so often if it brings your mood down. It's okay to vent a little, but what's the alternative—going back to the same lousy habits? Stay on target.

Plateaus are not unusual. During Scott's six months of intense weight loss, he experienced two plateaus. One lasted three weeks and one lasted four weeks. This slowing of weight loss can be very frustrating, but often that phase will end with a big drop in pounds.

As the days mount up during a plateau and there is no loss reflected on the scale, the temptation will be to give up and look in the mirror and say, "See, I told you so. I can't do this. Why did I think that I could ever succeed?" We have been right there with you. Exercise discipline and stay the course when you know you're being precise with your personal Diet Docs' Rx, power spacing, and food quality.

If you're not, it's not a plateau…it's a problem. Be honest with yourself and correct it. Don't give up now and experience a self-fulfilling prophecy. Joe told Scott, "Just stick with it, man. Stick with it." Scott felt like the guy in *Star Wars* flying down the trench in the Death Star with his commander telling him, "Stay on target, stay on target!" only to get barbecued by Darth Vader. He even thought about telling Joe where to "stick with it," but he believed in the program. He couldn't argue with his success so far and the success of others he had observed. Lo and behold, Scott did break through the plateaus and reach his goal. Hey, Joe was right! Well, duh! He's helped thousands of people lose thousands of pounds.

The reason you will smash through that plateau is because of the sound principles discussed in the earlier chapters. You are eating below the maintenance level of calories for your size so your body has no choice but to eventually relinquish some of your fat as fuel. Your fat cells are not like the shark in *Jaws*, stalking you, waiting for you to mess up. It is a biochemical reaction, and those little suckers won't have any choice but to shrink!

"I must have a slower metabolism than I thought."

Too many of us want to blame our metabolism for lack of weight loss. Metabolism is indeed important, but it's not at fault when we understand how to operate in the appropriate macronutritional range. If you haven't consumed enough nutrients, your metabolism will slow dramatically and you will have to work much longer and harder to lose weight. If you've consumed too much, you will gain weight. Chips and soft drinks have nothing to do with "slow metabolism." Focus on nutrition, discipline, health, and fun instead of the next creative rationalization.

"I'm too stressed to go on. I need a break."

This is one of the most difficult pitfalls to avoid. The first step in avoidance is preparation. Preparation against this problem comes in two forms. The first is by having plenty of healthy foods around so if you binge a little, you won't do too much damage. The second is to realize that you will binge eat due to stress at some point. Some people are fortunate enough to not eat (which is a problem unto itself) when they are stressed. However, many find comfort in chocolate or other things—that's why it's called "comfort food."

There may be times when stress eating starts, and you don't even realize it. You may be halfway through a pint of Häagen Dazs before you even know what hit you! As soon as you recognize you're eating due to stress, stop. You may be able to salvage the day and get back on track. You may go over just a bit but not lose your progress for the entire week. The only serious damage will be if you keep going.

Use the HALT method from Overeaters Anonymous. Think about why you are eating: *H*ungry or just *A*ngry, *L*onely, or *T*ired? Sometimes you may have to have a stare down with your food. You *can* walk away from that doughnut that's taunting you.

If stress eating is a big part of your life, deal with the issue. Don't underestimate the benefit of counseling. You are developing healthy mental discipline as well as physical discipline. Keep it up. Just as diet and exercise go hand in hand, so do the mental and physical portions of proper nutrition.

Life is life. Stress happens. Don't let it steamroll your health as well as your self-image. Stay in control. If you do let go of control, do two things. First, grab the reins back quickly. Second, get over it. Get back on track and let yesterday be yesterday. So what if you're not perfect 100 percent of the time? Will 85 to 90 percent be better than where you are now? You bet!

"I used to eat all my favorite foods and not gain a pound."

Don't you love the scene in *Freaky Friday* where the mind of the mother (Jamie Lee Curtis) is trapped in the teenage body of her daughter (Lindsay Lohan)? The mother's persona is savoring the french fries that she hasn't had for years. She can get away with it now that she's in her daughter's high-metabolism, 17-year-old frame. Don't we wish sometimes that we could go back to that? We wish we could eat whatever we want and not gain weight…like when we were 17.

There are several problems with this reasoning. First, some teenagers start getting fat on that type of diet before they get out of high school. In fact, this is even happening in grade school these days. We're teaching our kids incredibly poor nutrition habits that will carry into college and adulthood. When the metabolism starts to slow down (although it is a very slow decline), and when we don't get enough exercise, our abdomens begin to swell. As we age, it's much more the lack of movement than an actual decrease in basal metabolic rate that's the culprit for the supposed "decline" in metabolism.

We also have a hard time understanding we can't put away half a pizza and a 32-ounce soda like we did in college and still be okay. We trick ourselves into thinking that if we down that kind of fare we're still young and vigorous without a care in the world. If we eat like that, we couldn't possibly be getting old or fat, even though we have to spend the night with a bottle of Tums by our bedsides. Well, guess what? We *are* getting older, there *isn't* a fountain of youth, Ponce de Leon was just an ancient version of Ashton Kutcher with a funny metal helmet, and we've all been *punk'd*.

Retro snacking (thanks *Thirtysomething*) and eating junk will make us feel briefly nostalgic, but it also accelerates our demise. Proper nutrition and exercise, although not nearly so much fun initially, are the only ways toward healthy, vigorous lives. The ability to shoot hoops with your buddies or play with the kids when you're 45 is a lot more fun than standing on the sidelines.

Speaking for the male gender, men sometimes have the delusion that body mass equals health and dominance. "Hey, if I weigh 220 I must be the man!" No, all you are is bloated and sick. "The man" would suck it up and lose the extra weight. Being fit is being fit, and there are no shortcuts. You'll look a lot more like the cover of *GQ* at a lean, mean 170 than a puffy 220.

"It was just laying around. I *had* to eat it."

Don't be afraid to throw leftover junk food in the trash. Isn't your health worth more than half a bag of leftover chips that you *know* you'll eat if you leave it in your cabinet after a party? Why keep it around? For the kids? If you want to do something for kids, donate to St. Jude's or Jerry's Kids, but don't poison their little bodies with junk. And don't use that as an excuse for causing the premature death of their parents.

The Diet Docs' Rx, power spacing, and other structure provided in this book make dieting easier, but you *will* be faced with temptations of every kind. Don't make it a big, dramatic deal. Choose to walk away from that piece of cake or from the dinner table when you've had enough.

Planning ahead helps, but you can't prepare for everything other than knowing you'll face the food demons and need to walk away. Although it may be helpful to have a support group pat you on the back, you really don't need that for every triumph. Walk away because you *choose to do the right thing.*

"I eat when I'm depressed."

Some of us trace our need for comfort food back to our "trick or treat" days. We all have fond memories of getting treats as kids because that's exactly what they were—treats. We didn't get them every day or even every other day. But nowadays, as adults, we can jolly well eat whatever and whenever we want. But we have to learn to say no….or "HALT."

Before you put that bite in your mouth, ask if you're truly hungry or simply giving in to an emotion. Unfortunately for a lot of us, that "L" can also stand for "lazy" when we don't want to spend the time to prepare proper food or dispose of junk we don't need. Be practical. If you can't handle the bread basket at the restaurant table, tell the waiter not to bring it.

You spend a lot of money on a meal out, but you won't throw away 10-cents worth of half-eaten bologna? Think about it. You don't get a throwaway body. You have to take care of the one God gave you. Food is not an entitlement and neither is good health. Eating right is a sign of maturity and responsibility.

"I'm too undisciplined to stick with it."

"Discipline" isn't a bad word, although many of us are convinced it is. We're fiercely independent, and we don't like to be told we need to lose weight or exercise. Proverbs 5:23 tells us, "He will die for lack of discipline, led astray by his own great folly."

You don't want to die do you? Then learn the power of the word "no." You can create habits that will allow you to withstand the curve-balls life throws at you. These new habits help you get quickly back on track if you deviate. On a business trip? Say no to high-fat, high-carb foods until you can find a good option. If you honestly can't find anything healthy to eat, which we believe happens very rarely, control the amount you eat and get back on track with quality as soon as you can. There are no excuses for showing up at the airport with an empty briefcase when it could be loaded with healthy food.

The difference in a "cheat" meal and a "cheat" weekend is dramatic. We see so many people who diet during the week and then believe they can eat unrestrainedly over the weekend. And the weekend for them usually begins around noon on Friday and continues until Monday morning. So they're "dieting" barely 50 percent of the week, and the "eating normal" (which usually is not "normal" but excessive) doesn't allow them to lose weight.

Even at a ball park on a weekend you can make good choices. Have half a bottle of Gatorade, which may have a quarter of the carbs of a soda. Even better, carry a bottle of water. Take a protein bar with you. Eat a few peanuts, skip the cheeseburger, and eat when you get home. There are many, many options.

Bottom line: Self-discipline is enjoying doing what is right (within a flexible framework). Stop out-of-control eating. There are too many land mines in convenience foods in the forms of added sugar and fat. They are there to keep you hooked. If you're running to five different sports practices for your kids or working two jobs, you are a fast-food sales target. Be careful.

"I get tired of eating the same food."

You know what? Sometimes nutritious food and exercise are boring. There, we said it. But going to work every day can be boring, going to school can be boring...but you still do it.

Good health is *not* boring. Running with the kids for more than a minute isn't boring, playing tennis with your spouse isn't boring (exasperating but never boring), hiking outside and enjoying the world isn't boring, and living to see your great-grandchildren definitely isn't boring. Nutrition and exercise are the vehicles to get us there.

If absolutely necessary, take a vacation from strict dieting for a week. Increase your carbs by 25 to 50 grams a day, but still eat only *healthy* food. If you insist on taking a rebellious and total vacation from the diet, notice how you feel when you start eating poorly again. Use that feeling to stoke the desire to stay on track.

Cross-training is certainly a good thing when it comes to exercise, and the same can be applied to eating. Although most of us are creatures of habit, if you have wholeheartedly embarked on this journey of nutrition, you won't tire of learning new things. Consequently, keep looking for new options for fueling your body. Do the same with exercise. Tired of walking on a treadmill? Get on a bike or elliptical machine or take a kickboxing class. Tired of walking outside? Get an indoor exercise video to use during the winter months. Exercise and nutrition are not a burden; they are an incredible gift and blessing.

Rekindle the desire to work through the inevitable patches of boredom that strike. Take a break, but don't take a permanent vacation. Set new goals for your weight, exercise, and nutrition. Challenge yourself to stay motivated and fresh. Run with a friend in a local Race for the Cure or walk for March of Dimes. You can do it!

One of the important things about the Diet Docs' plan is that whether you are adventurous or like routine, you can do this diet. Variety is important for good nutrition, but if you like having the same thing every day, either way will work. To make sure you're not creating deficiencies, take a daily multivitamin.

If you're easily bored, experiment with variety. Try meats, vegetables, and fruits you haven't eaten in years. Since you aren't limited in the variety you can eat as long as you stay in your range, find some new, exciting foods that appeal to you.

Experimenting with protein shakes and bars, veggies, and dips make going to the grocery store fun, especially if you don't cook very much. Taking cooking classes with your spouse and learning about food and ingredients for dishes (they *do* make other things out of tomatoes than just ketchup) can be wonderful. If you don't like this kind of activity, eat whatever works for you. But remember, "variety" means making changes *within* a food group, such as vegetables. Fresh produce is an important part of any healthy diet. There is no way around that. Try different foods until you find what works and what you like and then lock in.

You sometimes have to do things you don't like to get healthy. Scott would love to walk around with one of those hats with a can of Mountain Dew on each side, a straw in his mouth, and a holster full of Pringles. But that won't get his blood pressure down, his lipids under control, or make his joints hurt any less. Joe would love to eat cheesecake until his thighs explode, but that won't help him keep up with his four rambunctious kids.

As you settle into the middle months of the plan, you'll find certain foods that help you stay on track. Although that can lead to a little bit of boredom, it can keep you focused and you will appreciate your splurge meals a lot more.

"My raging hormones won't cooperate with The Diet Docs' plan."

Lower levels of carbs over an extended period of time can lead to decreased testosterone and thyroid hormone. Scott definitely had a time with this when he dropped his carbs below what Joe recommended. These decreases in hormones can lead to feeling depressed. The way to combat that problem is to eat the recommended carbs in your personal Rx. Increase your carbs incrementally, as discussed in chapter 5, if you're losing too quickly. And try "cycling," raising and lowering your carbs during the week.

If you develop feelings of lethargy, increase your carbs slightly one or two days a week until the feeling passes. You may persist with that for a month or two until you get back on track. It's important you get these hormones back on line because you have to have the right frame of mind to stick with a healthy eating plan for the long haul.

Let's say, for example, that your carb intake should be 70 to 90 grams per day. You know you have the splurge meal on the weekend, so a good strategy to avoid feeling too carb depleted would be to stay close to 70 grams for 2 to 3 days, and then move up to 90 grams for a day. If you still have symptoms, such as feeling weak, fatigued, shaky, or lethargic, make sure your protein and fat are up to the maximum levels. Also change carb sources around a bit. Despite the glycemic index, some people do better on some carb sources than others.

"I'm too old. It's too late to change my habits now."

This may be one of the most legitimate pitfalls. Multiple aging problems, such as arthritis, sleep apnea, thyroid disease, heart medications, female hormone replacement, and diabetes, can lead to weight gain or difficulty in losing pounds. Even so, don't let this defeat you.

We have definitely seen many diabetics and patients on thyroid medication who have lost weight with this diet. Losing weight will help decrease back and arthritis pain and make diabetes and hypertension easier to control. Medication may make it harder to lose weight, but if you're still alive, your metabolism is still working, although its performance may not be optimal. Don't use medications or medical conditions as an excuse to quit working on nutrition and exercise. Realize that it may take longer to reach your goals, and you may have to modify your exercise program to fit your medical condition, but you can still be on this diet program. Once you're aware of your medication's side effects, work within the framework the medication allows.

If you're not making progress, discuss with your physician if there is an alternative prescription with fewer side effects. *Caution:* Many people don't want to take medication, and if you can use nutrition and exercise to discontinue your diabetes, hypertension, or cholesterol meds, that's great and is obviously a good goal. But *don't even think about doing that* until you've talked to your physician about what you want to do and why. Follow his or her advice!

Some medications may make you hungrier; but now you have the information to make good choices instead of opting for high-fat or high-carb foods. Comfort foods usually don't give us a lot of comfort as our bellies are pushing the rivets on our jeans to their maximum stress points. People in their mid-70s can lose weight. It can be done no matter what your age, with the proper supervision.

The bottom line is that it doesn't matter what age you are. People in their teens through their 80s have benefited from this program. You are never too old to learn about good nutrition, and teens can get it too.

"I get caught in social situations where I can't say no without seeming rude."

How can you tell Aunt Ella that you don't really want another slice of her sausage-and-beef pie with the cheese crust? Situations like this are guaranteed on vacation and even at work. You'll succeed a lot faster when you ditch the "Oh, what the heck, one won't hurt me" mentality.

Family, unfortunately, is often the worst about using that form of guilt. You wouldn't walk up to an alcoholic and say, "Oh, you've done so well the last few weeks. Here, have a drink." Avoid the habit of feeling obligated. You have to decide. Talk to your family members in advance and let them know that you don't want to hurt their feelings, but you're trying to lose weight. (Tell them you're on a healthy eating program, tell them you've been recruited by the Diet Docs... do whatever it takes.) Don't let them sabotage you with guilt. Smile politely and move on.

The same goes for coworkers. It's hard when someone brings in a treat and everyone is telling you how great it is. It's hard to walk away, but plan to do it. In Scott's little office of 15, there always seems to be a birthday, retirement, or special occasion. In a bigger office it could be even worse. Until you get yourself completely locked in, the polite but firm "No" will be your greatest weapon.

Dining out with friends—or even alone—can be tricky. Although some restaurants offer selections for diners watching their weight, many do not. Still, you *can* survive eating out if you're careful.

Surviving Restaurants

1. Specify how you want food prepared to avoid added butter, etc.

2. Order baked, grilled, or broiled entrees.

3. Ask for salad dressings on the side (fat-free, if possible).

4. Share a meal.

5. Ask for grilled or steamed veggies instead of a potato or rice to reduce carbohydrates.

6. Use red sauces instead of cream sauces.

7. Order a salad without cheese, croutons, bacon, egg yolks, and nuts.

8. Dip your fork in dressing and then your salad. You'll eat a lot less than pouring dressing on your salad.

9. Refuse complementary bread or chips.

10. Use a food nutrition count book to plan and estimate food intake.

11. Ask for a nutrition facts card/menu or go to the websites of your favorite restaurants so you have accurate information for your log book. That way you'll never be caught off guard.

"But I *deserve* it."

Watch out when you hear these words in your head! Overindulging after success can spin you back to failure. You can reward yourself in a regimented fashion, but be very careful. A sense of entitlement with food probably led to you overindulging in the first place. A moderate splurge meal once a week will give you something to look forward to and allow you to maintain your diet discipline.

We are all overworked and pressed for time, and that can lead us to the "reward" mentality. But you know what? Our parents and grandparents were overworked too. The major difference is they understood that hard work and sacrifice were part of daily living. They didn't have the money to reward themselves with a treat every time they did something, such as showing up for work and doing the job they were expected to do.

Getting up every day and doing the things we're supposed to do is a decent and honorable thing. But find a *better* reward than poisoning your body with junk food or portions so big your grandmother could have fed her entire family plus the nice couple next door.

"Working from home creates too much temptation."

Both our wives are work-at-home moms. Joe's wife has the benefit of living with someone who has made fitness a lifelong commitment. Scott's wife, on the other hand, has the burden of living with a slacker. And for moms and dads at home, the knowledge that a Dagwood-sized sandwich can be whipped up in ten minutes by raiding the fridge in the next room is a hard temptation to resist.

Work-at-home moms and dads face multiple diet problems: convenience, constant access to food, lack of time to exercise, and boredom.

Convenience is a problem all of us face whether it's stopping by the drive-through on the way home after gymnastics or giving a Pop Tart to the kids for breakfast while trying to get the oldest out the door and go over the middle child's spelling words. This is where shopping and prep time are very important. Make a double batch of a healthy entrée and freeze half of it. (Don't let it sit out and eat it!) Buy some low-fat peanut butter, berries, low-carb/low-fat yogurt. Change your kids' and your own eating habits. It only takes five minutes to eat a bowl of high-fiber cereal (trust us, we've timed it), so get up five minutes earlier and skip the doughnut at the office. Your health and your children's health are definitely worth five minutes.

At-home workers face the problem of "grazer mentality." Since they are in the kitchen a large percentage of the day—preparing meals, cleaning up, working on projects at the kitchen table with the little ones—they are constantly tempted to munch...and they only have to walk a few feet to have something. At work, there may be a constant supply of Krispy Kremes in the breakroom, sales reps with gift baskets, and a candy machine that's right on the way to the restroom. That bag of M&M's in the desk drawer will call your name often.

At home, if you find yourself glancing at the clock and feeling hungry, remember you have a meal or a healthy snack coming soon. You don't need to grab the junk. Don't nibble off your kids' plates (you wouldn't nibble off a coworker's plate would you?). You may need to change a few of your habits. Why not play board games in the living room instead of the kitchen? At work it's just as easy to keep dried fruit, nuts, and protein nuggets in your desk as that bag of candy that will leave you tired and run down.

Keep the fridge and the cupboards stocked with healthy food and get rid of the junk-food drawer. You are teaching your kids a lifetime of healthy eating and not depriving them of anything of value. We spend a lot of time teaching our children about priorities, sports, school, and life, so we don't want to neglect their health as well. Obviously it has to be age-appropriate, but teach them that there are important choices to be made in life about drinking, drugs, smoking, *and* eating.

One reason parents fail to discuss nutrition is the fear that we'll create eating disorders in our children. Concentrating on the health aspects and not only looks or physical appearance will help mitigate unhealthy eating patterns and thoughts. We also like to see our kids happy, and what lights them up more than candy or dessert? Another reason is fear of hypocrisy. It's hard to teach kids about good nutrition with chocolate chips wedged between your teeth.

There are great ways to work with your kids on nutrition. Since this book is about you, that's the focus. Your example, good or bad, is the most important impression you'll make on your children. Scott's girls actually came up to him and patted his stomach while saying they were glad he wasn't their fat daddy anymore. His son talked to him as Scott ran on the treadmill and then would hop on it when he was done. Scott says he cringes to think where his family would be if they hadn't started to address their health issues.

"My spouse isn't on board."

If your spouse isn't supportive, dieting can be a problem. As anyone can attest who tried to quit smoking when his or her spouse still puffed away, it is very difficult to quit. Trying to diet when your soul mate is eating cookies and ice cream after dinner and saying, "Mmm, mmm, good," is just plain hard. Some spouses will subconsciously sabotage a diet program because they believe they can't have the same kind of success the dieters are experiencing. Or they may fear that if their mates get in shape they will be a little too attractive to the opposite sex. Another problem may be they really don't want to have anyone telling them what to do. Or perhaps the pursuit of good health makes them feel guilty or dowdy.

The bottom line is that you are an adult. No one can control what goes in your mouth but you. If your partner sabotages your health, you will need to have a frank discussion about it. That's a *discussion*, not a fight. Reassure your sweetie that you want to be with him or her a long time and that is why you're taking better care of yourself. Have the quiet confidence to continue to eat right. Lead by example and respect the fact that your husband or wife may not be at the same point in his or her life. That is okay. Respect the difference. Don't badger your spouse into dieting. That must be his or her decision for the best outcome.

Scott's wife exercised for several years before he firmly got with the program. Any badgering by her launched him into an immature binge of getting a double scoop of rocky road and an "I'll show you" mentality. Over time he realized she loved him and just wanted to keep him around longer.

"I'm a rebel. Tell me I can't do something and I want to do it."

That nasty state of rebellion can derail any diet plan. No one wants to be told what to do. But if you're reading this, you probably want to be leaner, healthier, and feel better. Don't waste time on "Who the heck do these guys think they are?" statements. Maybe every once in a while it's okay to ask that. If you want to have one of those days—or even weeks—go right ahead. Notice how your intestines behave, what your energy level is like, what happens to your mental clarity, and what the scale does. If you have slid back into poor eating habits, you'll find that your body systems don't function nearly as well. Then you will remember why you decided to start eating in a healthy fashion. Use that independent streak to your advantage to get and stay healthy. Maybe you can change that "Born to Eat" tattoo to "Born to Eat Right."

"I feel uncomfortable when people talk about my weight loss."

It may sound strange, but some people are uncomfortable with compliments and the newfound attention they get from weight loss. Most of us welcome the positive attention, but if you're on the shy side it may seem easier to retreat into the shell of protection provided by extra weight. The weight sometimes allows you to "fly under the radar," which you may be more comfortable with.

There's a related danger that can be quite serious. If Scott is at a function and patients he's worked with on weight loss see him, they always bring up food. "I'm not eating that, Dr. Uloth, don't worry." "Oh, Dr. Uloth's here. Now I can't even eat that cookie I was going to have." And he feels the same pressure! How can he be a good example if he's caught publicly eating a brownie?

The splurge meal deals with this situation somewhat, and The Diet Docs' Rx provides flexibility that allows a little junk food at occasions like this if it fits into your daily food volume goals. The pressure of being seen "eating something bad" can entice us to be closet eaters. This is bad news. *Don't do it!* Joe jokingly loves to eat junk in front of clients to prove this point: in moderation, especially once you've reached your goals, a *small* variety of "nonhealth" food is normal and fun.

Another side to getting complimented is that success can become a pride issue. Scott tended to let people focus on *his* achievement rather than giving credit to his wife, Joe, and his commander-in-chief, God. Scott needed to take the focus off himself and back on the fact that his goal was about health and not just a certain look.

He remembers wishing it were a year down the road so all his patients would see "the new Dr. Uloth" and he could finally stop talking about it. Scott even entertained the notion that it might be a little easier if he gained some weight back so people wouldn't focus on it so much. However, he knew his health would suffer so he squashed that thought.

"I've blown it big time; I might as well give up."

The temptation to give up is a tremendous dieting pitfall. Two things happen with this thought pattern. We slip into a state of self-defeating behavior and continue to eat and eat. "Well, if I've already blown it, I might as well keep eating. I can't succeed at this weight loss thing anyway," we say, providing an excuse to indulge. When you're in a moderate calorie deficit and you start eating simple carbs, it's hard to stop. Your body will want more.

Psychologically, most of us contribute to backsliding with thoughts such as, *I might as well finish this off and get it out of my house,* or *I've been so good that this really won't set me back. I'll start again tomorrow.* Some people mistakenly think their bodies won't absorb much carbohydrate if they saturate themselves. Certainly your body can't use *all* those carbs, but it *will* absorb them and turn them into triglycerides to be stored as fat. Your body doesn't know the difference; it is simply built for survival. Your brain is the computer, so program it to tell your mouth when to stop. Develop a well-rehearsed emergency response plan to avoid a binge. You might drink a big glass of water, give yourself a quick pep-talk, or get away from the food. Surrender is not an option!

"But Dr. Atkins will let me eat…"

A diet that allows you to eat fat and protein as long as you eat no or low carbs only works in the short term for most people. Our program is designed for *permanent* weight loss…and that happens when the right amount of the macronutrients are consumed in moderate portions (based on The Diet Docs' Rx chart) and spaced appropriately.

"I work out regularly. Isn't exercise enough?"

This is one of the difficulties Scott ran into after he lost his excess weight and was in maintenance phase. It transpired about 10 months into the program, around the time of multiple birthday parties (his, his wife's, and his daughter's) and holidays (Halloween, Thanksgiving, and Christmas). He just couldn't forgo all those treats, and let's face it, what's better than a fun-size Snickers pilfered from your kids' trick-or-treat bag? He believed that since he was exercising regularly he could have a little dietary indiscretion and get away with it. A little turned into a lot, and before he knew it he'd gained 8 to 10 pounds. Scott kept saying he would "hit the diet hard" again after the first of the year, but with two weeks to go until New Year's, he realized he'd better get back on the wagon quickly before he gained 15 to 20 pounds!

Exercise is a cornerstone to any diet and physical fitness program, but exercise alone is not sufficient if you're eating high-fat, high-carb foods. Exercise will give you more freedom to enjoy yourself once in a while. It will give you the confidence of knowing you're in good shape and feel invigorated. The problem is that too many calories are shoved into small, convenient packages such as soda, chips, and candy that can stuff us with 600 to 700 calories in a matter of minutes without making us feel full. So don't go long stretches relying on exercise alone to keep you on your goal. Diet and exercise must go hand in hand. A weekend during the holidays is one thing, but if you go six weeks with an increasingly sporadic diet, you can do a tremendous amount of damage. You've worked too long and too hard to get here, so don't risk losing any of your progress.

A healthy dose of honesty is critical to success. After a not-so-great weekend of eating, my wife noted that the scale hadn't budged despite her routine exercise during those two days. She started to bemoan that fact and then stopped herself. She admitted, "I haven't done anything this weekend nutritionally to deserve the lower weight, so I'm not going to whine about it."

Pitfalls are out there. Even Indiana Jones isn't too old to find the treasure! Grab your whip, face the obstacles, and overcome them. Cue the John Williams music—ba ta dump da, ba da daaa…

Obstacles That Require Professional Help
Control Issues

Okay, let's pause to clarify something. Part of our job in this book is to help you regain control and give you hope. We want to help you get your out-of-control eating back to healthy by providing a solid framework so you won't feel like you're wandering alone in a vast desert of diet misfortune. For those of you who are control oriented, you'll need to loosen up a little and not crumble when you feel control over your nutrition slipping. Our program gives you flexibility. You don't have to be rigid with every meal and snack. *Lack* of flexibility often results in failure.

If your control issues are beyond that of the normal dieter…if your eating borders on or is at the magnitude of anorexia or bulimia, therapy is in order. Anorexia is far, far too complicated to blame it on our "diet-obsessed" culture and do nothing. People have been obsessed with their appearance since the ancient Egyptians came up with cosmetics. Eating disorders have nothing to do with good mental or physical health or proper nutrition. Anorexics pathologically believe that by controlling what goes into their bodies they can control their anxiety, obsessive-compulsive tendencies, lives, and what others think of them. These harmful, distorted beliefs can drive them to a destructive, and at times fatal, end. It is a devastating, incredibly hard illness that spirals out of control and is difficult to treat.

Eating disorders can consume entire families, and whatever can be done to combat these illnesses should take place. Saying "just eat more" to anorexics doesn't begin to address the pain these people (and their families) go through. Young people often don't realize that anorexia can lead to death from heart failure or arrhythmias from electrolyte abnormalities.

Equally disturbing is a trend we're seeing in adults who are undereating or overexercising in an effort to gain control of their lives. Sadly, far too often the eating disorder wins, and they and their families lose. If you (or someone you know) suffer from this illness, put this book down and seek help from a specialist trained in eating disorders. Often your family doctor or pediatrician is a good place to start, but he or she may not be adequately versed in providing long-term or follow-up care. The hardest step to take is realizing you're not in control, that your disorder is controlling you. If you've slipped near or past the edge of anorexia or bulimia, reach out right now! You need help, and you can be helped. Call your doctor right now.

Obesity can be just as devastating. Having a mother or father ripped from a family due to a heart attack, stroke, sleep apnea, or other problem leaves a family in ruin. Overeating to relieve stress or because we feel out of control is far more common than we think.

Morbid obesity may be a result of disordered thinking. We are saddened when a patient/client packs on weight as layers of protection against previous assaults. The assaults may have been sexual, physical, or verbal. These people believe the extra weight offers defense against unwanted sexual advances or makes them big and strong to stand up to a previous foe. The assailant from the past unfortunately often continues to inflict damage on his or her victim. If you are a victim of abuse or assault, please consider therapy. You can peel off the layers that threaten to destroy your physical and mental well-being. A good counselor will help you do this and feel safe.

If you want to lose weight but still have control issues, you'll have a hard time with permanent weight loss. The best thing you can do is deal with the control issue while beginning to work on weight loss. In rare cases, the control issue may need to be addressed before you begin a weight-loss program.

Key Points

1. Be patient; be prepared.

2. Trigger foods provoke strong emotions. Avoid them, especially in the first few weeks of your diet.

3. Plateaus are inevitable, but if you stay on target, you will break through!

4. Try something new. You're never too old.

5. A little hunger won't kill you.

6. Find a healthy way to relieve stress.

7. You must exercise and follow good nutrition to get and stay healthy.

The Diet Docs in Action...

Steve's Story

A few months after I turned 53 I got really tired of the fact that too many of my clothes were fitting tightly, even though I'd been jogging, riding my bike, and watching what I ate. The weight on my 5'6" frame just seemed to stay around 165 no matter what I did. This was 20 pounds more than I weighed just 10 years earlier. (I had lost 5 pounds on a popular plan when I was 50, but like almost everyone else I know who tried it, I had gained it all back.)

One day I happened to catch Dr. Joe on a local TV show. Having recognized him from church, I called him and set up an hour consultation. Joe's approach to nutrition and good body stewardship has affected my life dramatically. In fact, the change has been so dynamic in me it's a physical equivalent to the spiritual rebirth the Bible speaks of.

Dr. Joe simply gave me an eating plan to make my body start burning stored fat. Within 25 days I lost 10 pounds, and in less than 5 months I was down to 135. My weight has remained between 131 and 135 for 2 years—along with the 30" waist I had in high school. My energy and stamina multiplied. I feel like a new and different person! Medically speaking, my triglycerides have dropped from 249 to 88, my HDL ("good" cholesterol) rose from 46 to 68, and my LDL ("bad" cholesterol) dropped from 122 to 98.

On *The Diet Docs'* plan...

- I didn't get the munchies. I just got hungry for a meal of real food.

- I didn't feel like I was sacrificing anything food-wise.

- I didn't eat any "weird" food like rice cakes or celery bread or grapefruit rind.

- I wasn't hungry for the cookies, cake, pie, etc., that had been one of my "basic food groups" all my life. It didn't bother me to pass by the many sweets that I frequently encounter during the course of a day.

- I don't have any plan or desire to go back to my old eating habits. I love/enjoy what I'm eating now and could eat this way for the rest of my life.

continued ➤

With the newfound energy that intelligent eating gives me, I'm able to do a vigorous workout 3 times a week. At 55, I am in the best shape of my life! Last year I set personal lifetime speed records for running the 5K, and was also able to climb 5,235 feet to the ridge crest of Mt. Whitney (13,600 ft.) and back in one day.

I have come to realize that an hour of vigorous exercise is not a waste of time "when you should be doing something more important." It is tuning up your body so you can accomplish in a more efficient way what God needs you to. The hour I spend lifting weights or running I get back in the one less hour of sleep I need, a more alert mind, and a relaxed body.

I know that there are many weight-loss theories and programs; however, I can't help thinking there is something very unique and permanent about The Diet Docs' approach. And you won't find anyone with a keener mind who is more concerned about your total well-being than Dr. Joe. The surge in my self-confidence that he gave me has resulted in positive effects too numerous to mention. Thanks a million, Joe!

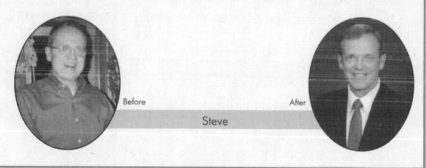

Before   After

Steve

CHAPTER 12

Keeping Excess Weight Off Forever

There's nothing more disheartening than to gain back a significant portion of the weight you lost by working diligently to lose it. You may already know this from past experience. It's called yo-yo dieting for obvious reasons. This can be a thing of the past for you—if you break the old pattern of bad habits and apply what you've learned in this book.

Some of the blame for yo-yo dieting lies at the foot of physiology. If your previous diets included a severe decrease in carbohydrates or insufficient calories, your metabolic rate may have suffered significantly. Once a higher food intake was reestablished, you may have regained body fat rapidly until your metabolic rate rebounded. By then it was too late. That's one danger of a very low-calorie or low-carb diet. The wildly fluctuating blood sugar spins you into levels of hunger you aren't used to. Before you know it, you're eating an incredible amount of carbohydrates and converting a large portion of them into body fat *again*. This is the exact cycle you bought this book to avoid.

A second reason for failure, and often in conjunction with the first, is letting your guard down and not adjusting your food choices properly. If you were to plow through a few days of really high-carb intake, especially of the typical binge or "celebration" foods, it's very hard to recover. And you may know that by bitter experience. So how do you change this pattern?

Once you reach your desired weight goal, bring your food intake up to a maintenance level where you will no longer lose weight but also not gain any. You won't raise your protein levels; they've already been set to give you an ideal amount. However, fat and carbohydrates may be raised in tandem but not necessarily in equal amounts. You may find that 10 to 15 extra grams of fat and 25 extra grams of carbs will provide enough energy and calories. If this slows your rate of loss but doesn't stop it completely, take another step upward…and then another until maintenance is reached.

Many important things will happen by making this process incremental. First, your blood chemistry will remain more stable, and you'll be less likely to experience binge-causing hunger due to the increase in carbohydrates. Second, you'll slowly rebuild any decreases in your metabolic rate that may have occurred due to the length of your diet. This will help ensure you won't regain body fat. As a matter of fact, you'll find you have to slowly keep adding more food to not lose weight. The amount of carbohydrates and fat you add is entirely up to you, but keep several health and behavioral points in mind.

You still want to adhere to the same health-building habits you've created through The Diet Docs' Plan. Keep good fats in your diet and keep saturated fats low. Stick with low-glycemic index carbs as much as you can. If you maintain these principles, your increase in food will leave you with high energy, stability, and controlled weight. Experiment with different levels of carbohydrates and fat to find your best maintenance level of food.

You may operate better with one macronutrient raised disproportionately to the other. This has to do with metabolic body type. An insulin-sensitive person may get hungrier on a higher level of carbs and tend to gain weight back. However, with carbs remaining a little lower and fat increasing, the same person may have no hunger, high energy, and no weight gain. A person fortunate enough to have a high metabolism tends to be an "ectomorph"—able to consume a higher percentage of calories from carbs without weight gain. Beware, though. Despite being able to get away with more carbs, an ectomorph can still gain weight.

One last point: As you transition into maintenance, you're exiting a dieting level of food that includes less carbs than your body needs for energy. As you increase your food, you will be refilling your liver and muscles with a higher amount of glycogen. Glycogen attracts and holds water. You will undoubtedly gain a couple of pounds due to water, just as the first couple of pounds you lost were water weight. Don't be alarmed; this is normal hydration and a normal level of carbohydrates stored in your body.

Make sure you don't gain more than a couple pounds once you've hit your lowest weight. Your body-fat level won't be affected; the weight will be water and glycogen. This is another reason to keep your upward changes slow and incremental. You don't want to fret over water gain, but you also don't want to be deceived into thinking you're gaining just water when it may be fat.

So there you have it. If patiently and carefully handled, the transition into maintenance will be smooth and successful. Instead of regaining weight you can experience an increasing level of energy, an increasing metabolic rate, and control of your weight.

That, after all, is your goal!

The Diet Docs in Action...
Sally and Paul's Story

I have struggled with my weight since I was in my late 20s after I delivered our daughter, Sarah. Each year I gained a few pounds, until at 49 years of age I weighed over 200 pounds. Because weight was such an issue in my family growing up, I'd sworn off all diets. I didn't really eat a lot of food, but I was eating all the wrong foods. But, during all those years, I continued exercising three to five times a week—walking, riding my bike, swimming, tennis, etc. So for a heavy woman I was in fairly good shape.

Paul, as a farmer, was always very active. He, like me, was gaining a few pounds each year. His doctor told him he needed to lose weight, especially since his cholesterol was high.

In 2003 I was student teaching the first half of the year and beginning a new position at the University of Southern Indiana as a math instructor the second half of the year. I was so busy I had no time to exercise or cook. At least two to three times a week we went out to eat fast food—cheeseburgers, french fries, and soda—food I never thought I could live without. Because I wasn't able to exercise, my weight ballooned to 218. By December 2003, I was experiencing a lot of knee pain and shoulder pain. I was also very tired and sick of living like this. I was finally ready to change my eating habits.

We'd heard about Dr. Joe and his eating plan two years prior. I e-mailed him and set up an appointment in January. I knew that if I didn't do it then, I wouldn't feel like it in January. I remember going to that first appointment thinking, *What am I doing? I am still so snowed under from my job I can't put any effort into this now.* But I also knew that if I didn't do it now, I wouldn't do it later.

Paul agreed to go with me, knowing that he needed to lose too. He didn't want to go on any diet because he was afraid we would just gain it back.

We met with Dr. Joe, and he explained the physiology of eating and losing weight. I had told myself that, yes, I needed to lose weight, but more importantly I needed to learn how to eat right. Dr. Joe gave us each our plan of right eating—the amount of protein, carbs, and fat we should eat each day and how to put them together. Then he sent us home to implement it. We ate our last fast-food dinner and went to bed.

continued ⟶

We got up the next morning and looked at each other—where do we begin? We were totally clueless on the nutritional value of food. The first few days (and weeks) were difficult as we struggled to put our foods together and stay under the prescribed amount of protein, carbs, and fat. I started a spreadsheet to help us add up our grams each day. We soon realized that starting at dinner and planning backward was the key for us. The eating plan allowed us the freedom to eat what we like…within reason. It didn't stop us from eating out or eating with our friends. It just gave us the tools and the information we needed to make our eating healthy and fit our likes and dislikes.

Every Wednesday morning Paul and I would weigh in front of each other and mark our progress. We still do that to this day. The eating plan worked like clockwork. Each week I lost about one to one-and-a-half pounds and Paul would lose one-and-a-half to two pounds. By the end of May, Paul had lost 50 pounds, meeting his goal of 175. I continued on, losing 75 pounds by the middle of October and meeting my goal of 145. As I began eating better, I also began training to walk/run a minimarathon in Indianapolis.

By April I had lost 35 pounds and finished the minimarathon in less than 3 hours. By October I was down to my goal weight and participated in my second minimarathon in Evansville and finished in just over two-and-a-half hours.

Paul continues farming and working outside each day.

We both feel so much better. My knees and shoulders don't hurt anymore. We both have more energy and love being able to go into any store and buy clothes without trying them on. I used to wear a size 22, but now I wear a size 10. Paul went from a size 38 to a size 34. Our eating plan has become a change of life for us. We will never look at food the same. We don't always eat like we should, but we keep close tabs on our weight and adjust our eating to match. Many people have followed The Diet Docs' plan after seeing what we were able to do.

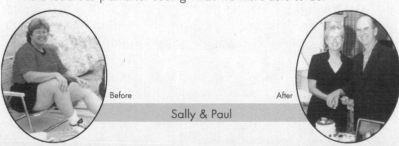

Before   After

Sally & Paul

CHAPTER 13

Food Prep
& Recipes

Just Tell Me What to Eat!

Most new clients sit across from Joe in full trust, expecting body-fat loss and positive health changes similar to what they've seen in the person who referred them. Occasionally someone helps us by offering feedback on the information or methods of delivery. We've learned a great deal and invite any criticism and feedback you want to share. But there is one common request we always refuse. A mild version of this request is a client who asks for recipes and meal plans and then hints at wanting an entire daily menu. The more severe version comes from clients who beg for a written menu to follow or they believe they simply won't succeed. They say, "I promise, just tell me what to eat and I'll eat it! I don't care if I eat the same thing every meal, every day."

For these clients, we predict failure. They usually have tried everything else and failed more as a result of lacking initiative and discipline than faulty nutrition plans. Sorry to be so blunt, but keep reading and you'll understand.

Though it may seem easier, you really don't want to follow a meal-by-meal plan written by us…or anyone else. Nobody knows what foods you like, what your schedule is, and what challenges are unique to you. You need to learn to interact with food—any food— in a healthy way so you can incorporate good foods into your daily plan successfully. For the sake of reference and to start you with some ideas, we will provide a small number of meals for you to view as examples. But the goal is for you to create your own food intake based on the nutritional values proposed in chapter 5.

If you came to Joe through a class, a consultation, or his on-line program, he would purposely make the first step personal menu planning. You'd then go home and figure out what you were going to eat the next day, making the best food choices, keeping nutrient totals and meal spacing as even as possible, and creating four to six meals that fall into your personal Diet Docs' Rx.

Yes, it takes a food count book, a calculator, an eraser, and a lot of patience. Once you've taken this step, however, you're well on your way to success because you have a framework from which to build a pattern. You will quickly learn to substitute a variety of food and meal choices and stay within your plan. Without this planning, you probably won't continue the diet successfully. The responsibility is yours. You become the driving force that makes the nutritional elements work in your daily life. You learn to adapt, be creative, and step out on an ongoing journey of learning. You become your own nutritionist. *You* succeed.

Many people who join a weight-loss center end up gaining back most, all, or more than the lost weight within one year. These weight-loss centers pride themselves on making it easy for their customers by providing diet plans, meal cards, follow-along daily menus, and even prepackaged food. On this issue, we gladly walk in the opposite direction.

The initial ease offered by set menus is quickly complicated by the fact that you have a different schedule, different tastes, different goals, and different metabolic needs than everyone else. Second, you learn little about nutrition and how to make permanent changes. Our plan is a little more difficult and time consuming on the front end, but the information will stick in your brain and make it easier to follow for the rest of your life. No one can take this knowledge away from you and no program is waiting for you to return and spend more money.

What's That?

Many successful clients have suggested we write a recipe book. Maybe someday we will, but for now we've included this recipe section to get you started. Along with the meal samples provided, you now have enough food information to create innumerable days of good meals within your personal Rx. And that's what it's all about: using foods you like to merge "natural" eating habits into the ranges that will accomplish your goal.

Check out the bookstore or library for full recipe books that suit your taste and the type of meal ratios you're looking for. There are books that cater to lower-carb meals, lower-fat meals, or whatever you need help with in structuring your menus. Begin with the understanding that eating the right foods in the right amounts at the best times is your focus. You don't have to make a meal for your family and a separate meal for yourself. You don't have to have elaborate recipes and exotic ingredients or even "special" foods to eat healthily. Right foods, right amounts.

You can throw a can of tuna in a bowl with a cup of brown rice, stir in a half a tablespoon of flaxseed oil, pour on some salsa, and you're ready to eat.

Breakfast? No problem! Mix a scoop of strawberry protein powder into an already-cooked half-cup of oatmeal, add some almonds or oil, and you're off to the office. Creativity! You may get some funny looks once in a while, but you'll have the last laugh. Scott got some snickers as he chomped on his ostrich jerky (one of his favorite snacks), but he lost 60 pounds!

When you put this book down, take a tour of your kitchen and look at the three macronutrient categories on the food labels. Some will pleasantly surprise you, and some will spur you to put green Poison Control Center stickers on the boxes.

Now you're taking an active role in your nutrition.

Breakfast Without Sugar

Most breakfast selections are a disastrous way to start your day. Sugar and refined (high-glycemic) flour are used to create tasty cereals—as long as you don't mind a little extra body fat, low energy, and hunger. You're not a cereal person? How about a doughnut or a "healthier" refined-flour bagel with 50 grams of carbs? Breakfast bars, pastries—yep, same story.

Breakfast is actually a difficult meal for most people due to time constraints and/or a lack of food ideas. Unless you want the tuna and salsa concoction for breakfast, pay attention. Protein in the morning is difficult unless you plan ahead. Take time to cook egg white combinations or utilize a protein substitute. Scrambled egg whites (with one whole egg if you like and if the extra fat fits in your meal plan) cooked in olive or canola oil, joined by oat or rye toast, make a great breakfast. You can even get fancy with different omelets. Check out Figure 13.1 just before the Recipe section for more ideas.

Oatmeal (watch for added sugar in flavored brands) is an excellent choice and can be fortified with good fat and protein such as half a scoop of protein powder and almonds. Meal replacement shakes are also very helpful. These are protein powders packaged in individual servings (or large canisters). These products make great shakes in a blender. You can add your choice of high-quality oil and low-glycemic fruit if you choose to "spend" that amount of carbohydrate at breakfast. You can't get much quicker than that.

One idea that may help you decrease your reliance on huge amounts of processed carbs at breakfast is to view it as just another meal. Bodybuilders will sometimes eat yet another chicken breast and green beans for breakfast (gross!). You don't need to go to that extreme, but who said we need eight ounces of juice and a stack of pancakes for breakfast? It's an important meal to not skip, but try increasing your protein and decreasing your carbs. You'll be less hungry later, and you'll have more energy. Plus you will save more carbs for later meals and snacks. That's all good!

Lunch and Supper the Easy Way

Lunch and supper, or even whole food snacks, can easily be pieced together by combining compatible protein, carbohydrate, and fat choices. Choose your protein source first and then add complementary carbs and fat. If it's a chicken breast, decide whether you want pasta, brown rice, a sweet potato—your choice. Add a limited amount of a healthy fat (if necessary to reach your suggested nutrient totals). Eat with confidence. A deli (chicken or turkey breast) sandwich can be made with low-glycemic bread and condiments. Health food stores even have mayonnaise made with canola oil instead of saturated fat. A chicken breast salad with a little Italian dressing is a great option. The salad vegetables give you great carbs and the dressing gives you olive oil. Your creativity and planning are the only factors keeping you from enjoying great tasting food and easy-to-prepare meals. Check out Figure 13.2 just before the Recipe section for menu examples.

Snacks

Snacks are vital to your plan. They keep your blood chemistry stable (as long as your food choices are appropriate), lessen hunger, help prevent overeating at meals, and keep metabolism high. Convenience can compromise quality if you're not careful though. To keep food quality high, snacks may be an area where you need to be more flexible with the spacing of your nutrients.

For example, an apple and an eighth of a cup of almonds make a great snack of low-glycemic carbs and quality fat, but the protein is low. Making sure your protein was adequate at your previous and your next meals is, therefore, imperative. There are also a few high-quality snack bars that have a balanced amount of protein, carbs, and fat. They are especially good when you crave chocolate or a treat since there are many great flavors out there. Bars come in many sizes so stick to the right amount for your meal or snack even if you have to eat half and save the rest for later.

After-dinner snacks can consist of a small amount of carbs or a protein shake. (Keep your eyes on those serving sizes. A microwave bag of popcorn is three servings!) Try to keep under 150 to 200 calories per late-night snack. Look at Figure 13.3 just before the Recipe section for examples.

Weight loss will be accelerated if after-dinner snacking is eliminated or minimized, so be vigilant. If you eat a protein-only snack at night, you'll decrease sleeping levels of insulin and your body will release more growth hormone, which increases recovery from exercise and also speeds fat loss. Joe often has a scoop of protein powder, and with some creativity in preparation it becomes like dessert. For example, a scoop of banana-flavored protein powder with a tiny amount of water in a bowl whipped with a fork into a cake frosting consistency with half a graham cracker crumbled in: It tastes just like vanilla wafer banana pudding!

Simple Breakfasts

Food Source	Protein	Carbs	Fat
3 egg whites	12	0	0
1 piece whole grain toast	2	13	1
1 tsp. canola oil (to cook eggs)	0	0	4
Total	14	13	5

(A great light breakfast that is very balanced and filling.)

Food Source	Protein	Carbs	Fat
6 egg whites/1 yolk	27	0	6
2 pieces whole grain toast	4	26	2
1 tsp. canola oil	0	0	4
Total	31	26	12

(Similar breakfast but larger.)

Food Source	Protein	Carbs	Fat
1/2 cup (dry) oats	5	27	3
1 scoop protein powder	30	5	1
1/2 tbsp. flaxseed oil	0	0	6
Total	35	32	10

Mix powder and oil into oats after oats are cooked.

(Protein powder is optional but does significantly fortify this already great breakfast.)

Food Source	Protein	Carbs	Fat
1/2 cup low-fat cottage cheese	13	4	5
4 egg whites	16	0	0
1 tsp. canola oil (to cook eggs)	0	0	4
Chopped omelet veggies	0	3	0
Total	29	7	9

Mix cottage cheese and egg whites in bowl, and then make omelet.

(A high-protein, low-carb breakfast that is versatile and tastes great. Add carb sources, such as toast, if desired.)

Figure 13.1

Simple Breakfasts cont.

Food Source	Protein	Carbs	Fat
¹/₂ cup low-fat, plain yogurt	8	10	2
1 scoop protein powder	30	5	1
¹/₈ cup almonds	3	3	7
¹/₄ cup (dry) oats	3	13	1
Total	44	31	11

Mix everything together into yogurt. May substitute high-fiber cereal for oats. Add fruit for more carbs if needed. Cut ingredients in half if necessary for your meal plan. (This quick option tastes like dessert for breakfast!)

Food Source	Protein	Carbs	Fat
Meal replacement shake	40	20	1
¹/₂ tbsp. flaxseed oil	0	0	5
8 oz. skim milk	8	4	2
Total	48	24	8

May substitute 1 tbsp. peanut butter for flaxseed oil. May use water instead of milk. Blend in mixer with ice. May use scoop of protein powder instead of meal replacement packet to decrease protein and carbs. (This is a quick but significant jump-start for the day.)

Food Source	Protein	Carbs	Fat
1 cup high-fiber cereal	3	35	1
1 cup skim milk	8	4	2
¹/₂ scoop protein powder	15	2	1
Total	26	41	4

Mix vanilla protein powder in milk and pour on cereal. (You can't get breakfast much faster than this, but measure well; the carbs in cereal add up fast!)

Food Source	Protein	Carbs	Fat
3 egg whites	12	0	0
2 pieces low-fat turkey bacon	6	0	2
1 tsp. canola oil (for cooking)	0	0	4
2 pieces whole grain toast	4	26	2
Total	22	26	8

May use whole grain pancakes instead of toast. May drop 1 piece of toast to decrease carbs. May make into sandwich. (If you have time, this is a classic!)

Figure 13.1 cont.

Lunch and Dinner

Food Source	Protein	Carbs	Fat
5 oz. chicken breast	35	0	5
1/2 cup rice	2	22	0
Salad or can of green beans	0	10	0
2 tbsp. low-/no-fat dressing	0	2	2
Total	37	34	7

(This is a full-size lunch or supper complete in all categories.)

Food Source	Protein	Carbs	Fat
4 oz. deli turkey breast	28	0	4
2 pieces whole grain bread	4	26	2
Lettuce/tomato	0	3	0
Mustard	0	0	0
Total	32	29	6

May use 1 piece of bread to decrease carbs and add a small salad to increase fiber. (A plain ol' sandwich can be a great meal.)

Food Source	Protein	Carbs	Fat
4 oz. tuna	30	0	0
1 tbsp. light mayo	0	2	3
Small salad	0	10	0
5 small whole wheat crackers	0	10	2
Total	30	22	5

(Quick and easy tuna salad.)

Food Source	Protein	Carbs	Fat
3 oz. chicken breast strips	21	0	3
1 tortilla wrap	0	5	1
Lettuce, veggie condiments	0	5	0
3 to 4 tbsp. salsa	0	5	0
Total	21	15	4

(Creative and delicious!)

Food Source	Protein	Carbs	Fat
Chicken breast sandwich/sub	30	35	5

Estimate well or look up in a food count book. Ask for no mayo, no cheese. (Everyone's on the go sometimes!)

Figure 13.2

Lunch and Dinner cont.

Food Source	Protein	Carbs	Fat
Meal replacement shake made with water	40	20	1
(Not the preferable whole food lunch, but quick in a pinch.)			
Protein bar	30	30	7
(Best used as a snack so you get fiber and whole food meals, but in an emergency…)			
Small salad	0	10	0
1/2 cup low-fat cottage cheese	13	4	5
Pop-top can of chicken	13	0	1
Total	26	14	6
(Just a quick, small lunch option.)			
4 oz. baked fish	24	0	1
1 cup steamed broccoli	0	8	0
4 oz. baked potato	1	30	0
1 tsp. butter	0	0	5
Total	25	38	6
(A great pattern for dinner.)			
1/2 oz. almonds	3	3	6
3 oz. chicken	21	0	3
1 tbsp. light mayo	0	2	3
Dash of curry (spice)	0	0	0
2 pieces whole wheat bread	6	24	0
Total	30	29	12
(Any recipe can be used as long as the amounts of foods used are measured and tracked. Be creative!)			

Figure 13.2 cont.

Snacks on the Run

Food Source	Protein	Carbs	Fat
Meal replacement shake made with water	40	20	1
Protein bar	30	30	7
1 scoop protein powder	30	5	0
½ cup skim milk	4	5	0
½ cup pineapple	0	15	0
1 cup strawberries	1	11	0
1 tsp. flaxseed oil	0	0	4
Total	35	36	4

(Add ice, blend, freeze, and thaw out about one hour before eating. Tastes like frozen yogurt. Or just blend and drink!)

Food Source	Protein	Carbs	Fat
½ cup skim milk	4	5	0
½ scoop protein powder	15	2	0.
1 tbsp. peanut butter	5	4	8
Total	24	11	8

(You can make an infinite variety of protein shakes.)

Food Source	Protein	Carbs	Fat
Energy/snack bar	16	24	8
Apple	1	30	0

(Yep, just an apple can be fine. Watch out though. As a stand-alone carb source you may get hungry soon after.)

Food Source	Protein	Carbs	Fat
Yogurt (low or fat free)	10	20	3

Figure 13.3

Sugar Saving Substitutions

Several sugar substitutes exist and may be used to replace sugar sources in cooking, baking, and general sweetening. Though tastes are individual, most artificial sweetener packets can replace two teaspoons of sugar. Noncalorie sweeteners include stevia, aspartame (Equal), saccharin (Sweet 'N Low), acesulfame K, and sucralose (Splenda). Our recommendation is stevia, an almost noncaloric sweetening agent derived from a cactus-like plant.

Sugar	Substitutes (packets)	Substitutes (bulk)
2 teaspoons	1 packet	$^1/_2$ teaspoon
$^1/_4$ cup	6 packets	3 teaspoons
$^1/_3$ cup	8 packets	4 teaspoons
$^1/_2$ cup	12 packets	6 teaspoons
$^3/_4$ cup	18 packets	9 teaspoons
1 cup	24 packets	12 teaspoons

Recipes

Breakfast

Cheese Omelet, 213

Country Scrambled Eggs, 213

Dilly Scrambled Eggs, 214

Oat Waffles, 214

Spinach Egg Bake, 215

Veggie Omelet, 216

Lunch

Broccoli Cheddar Soup, 217

Chicken Cheddar Wraps, 218

Garden Tuna Sandwiches, 218

Italian Mushroom Salad, 219

Mushroom Turkey Burger, 220

Soft Chicken Tacos, 220

Spinach Chicken Wraps, 221

Vegetarian Burritos, 222

Dinner

Blueberry Chicken, 223

Broccoli–Cabbage Slaw, 224

Cajun Salmon Steaks, 224

Chicken Burritos, 225

Chicken Veggie Stew, 226

Chili Chicken Breasts, 227

Cilantro–Lime Cod, 227

Creamed Mushroom Turkey, 228

Creamy Chicken Enchiladas, 229

Creamy Pea Salad, 230

Curry Chicken Breasts, 231

Dill Salmon, 231

Garlic Chicken, 232

Herbed–Lime Chicken, 233

Italian Chicken Cutlets, 234

Italian Orange Roughy Fillets, 234

Italian–Tomato Chicken, 235

Lean and Meaty Spaghetti Sauce, 236

Lean Swedish Meatballs, 236

Lemon Baked Salmon, 237

Lemon Chicken, 238

Lemon Fish, 239

Light Spinach Quiche, 239

Light Turkey Salad Tortillas, 240

Mini Turkey Loaves, 241

Mushroom Spinach Tart, 242

Orange Roughy Primavera, 243

Oriental Sesame Chicken, 244

Parmesan Chicken, 244

Southwest Chicken, 245

Spicy Haddock, 245

Spicy White Chili, 246

Stuffed Sole, 247

Sweet and Spicy Chicken, 248

Turkey Tortilla Pie, 248

Zesty Cod, 249

Recipes
(continued)

Dessert

Blueberry Pie, 250

Cherry Cream Pie, 251

Chocolate Mousse, 251

Creamy Raspberry Pie, 252

Eggnog Pudding, 253

Lemon Blueberry Cheesecake, 253

Lemon Mousse, 254

Light Carrot Cake, 255

No-Bake Chocolate Cheesecake, 256

Orange Whip, 257

Peanut Butter Pudding, 257

Pear Squares, 258

Pumpkin Spice Dip, 259

Breakfast

Cheese Omelet

4 egg whites
¼ teaspoon onion powder
¼ teaspoon dried basil
¼ teaspoon dried parsley flakes
¼ teaspoon celery seed
¼ cup fat-free shredded cheddar cheese

In a bowl beat egg whites and seasonings.

Lightly coat skillet with cooking spray and heat skillet. Add egg mixture. Cook over medium heat. As eggs set, lift edges, letting uncooked portion flow underneath. When eggs are completely done, remove from the heat. Place cheese over half of the eggs. Fold over other half and serve.

Yield: 1 serving

Nutritional analysis: One serving equals 118 calories, 2 grams (g) fat, 6 g carbohydrate, 19 g protein

Diabetic exchanges: 2 meat/cheese

Country Scrambled Eggs

12 egg whites, 2 yolks
¾ cup diced, fully cooked ham
¾ cup fat-free shredded cheddar cheese
½ cup chopped fresh mushrooms
¼ cup chopped onion

In a bowl beat eggs. Add ham, cheese, mushrooms, and onion.

Lightly coat skillet with cooking spray and add egg mixture. Cook and stir over medium heat until eggs are completely set and cheese is melted.

Yield: 4 servings

Nutritional analysis: One serving equals 134 calories, 6 g fat, 4 g carbohydrate, 16 g protein

Diabetic exchanges: 1½ meat/cheese, 1 fat, ½ vegetable

Dilly Scrambled Eggs

6 egg whites, 2 yolks
¼ cup skim milk
Dash of pepper
Cheese, shredded
1 teaspoon snipped fresh dill or ¼ teaspoon dill weed

In a bowl beat the eggs, milk, and pepper. Lightly coat skillet with cooking spray and heat. Add egg mixture. Cook and stir gently over medium heat until eggs are almost set. Sprinkle with cheese and dill. Cook until eggs are completely set and cheese is melted.

Yield: 2 servings

Nutritional analysis: One serving equals 139 calories, 7 g fat, 3 g carbohydrate, 16 g protein

Diabetic exchanges: 1½ meat/cheese, 1 fat

Oat Waffles

1 cup all-purpose flour
1 cup oat flour
4 teaspoons baking powder
3 egg whites

1¾ cups skim milk
2 tablespoons canola oil
1 teaspoon vanilla extract

In a bowl combine the first 3 ingredients.

Combine the egg whites, milk, oil, and vanilla. Stir into dry ingredients until just combined. Pour batter by ½ cupful into a preheated waffle iron. Bake until golden brown.

Yield: 8 waffles

Nutritional analysis: One waffle equals 147 calories, 3 g fat, 24 g
carbohydrate, 6 g protein

Diabetic exchanges: ½ meat/cheese, ½ milk, ½ fat, 1½ starch

Spinach Egg Bake

1 cup seasoned bread crumbs
2 packages (10 ounces *each*) frozen chopped spinach, thawed and
squeezed dry
3 cups (24 ounces) small-curd, fat-free cottage cheese
½ cup grated, fat-free Parmesan cheese
8 egg whites, 2 yolks

Sprinkle ¼ cup bread crumbs into a nonstick cooking spray-coated 8-inch square baking dish. Bake at 350 degrees for 3 to 5 minutes or until golden brown.

In a bowl combine the spinach, cottage cheese, Parmesan cheese, 6 egg whites, 1 yolk, and remaining crumbs.

Spread mixture over the baked crumbs.

Beat remaining 2 egg whites and 1 yolk. Pour over spinach mixture.

Bake uncovered at 350 degrees for 45 minutes or until a knife inserted near the center comes out clean. Let stand for 5 to 10 minutes before serving.

Yield: 4 servings

Nutritional analysis: One serving equals 176 calories, 4 g fat, 15 g carbohydrate, 20 g protein

Diabetic exchanges: 1½ meat/cheese, 1 starch, 1 vegetable, ½ fat

Veggie Omelet

¼ cup diced green pepper
¼ cup diced onion
¼ cup sliced mushrooms
4 egg whites
Pinch of pepper
2 tablespoons fat-free shredded cheddar cheese

In an 8-inch skillet sauté green pepper, onion, and mushrooms in nonstick cooking spray until tender. Remove and set aside.

In a small bowl beat egg whites, salt, and pepper. Pour into a skillet. Cook over medium heat. As eggs set, lift edges, letting uncooked portion flow underneath. When the eggs are completely set, spoon vegetables and cheese over one side and fold rest of eggs over filling. Cover and let stand for 1 to 2 minutes or until cheese is melted.

Yield: 1 serving

Nutritional analysis: One serving equals 98 calories, 2 g fat, 3 g carbohydrate, 17 g protein

Diabetic exchanges: 1½ meat/cheese, 1 vegetable

Lunch

Broccoli Cheddar Soup

1 large bunch broccoli, coarsely chopped (5 cups)
2 tablespoons cornstarch
2 cups skim milk
1 cup chicken broth
1 tablespoon canola oil-based butter
¼ teaspoon salt
⅛ teaspoon pepper
1 cup (8 ounces) shredded fat-free cheddar cheese
Dash of paprika

In a saucepan bring 1 inch of water to a boil. Place broccoli in a steamer basket over water. Cover and steam for 5 to 8 minutes or until crisp-tender.

In another saucepan combine the cornstarch, milk, and broth. Beat until smooth. Bring to a boil. Cook and stir for 2 minutes or until thickened. Stir in the butter, salt, and pepper. Reduce heat. Add cheese and broccoli. Heat until cheese is melted. Sprinkle with paprika and serve.

Yield: 4 servings

Nutritional analysis: One serving equals 123 calories, 3 g fat, 17 g carbohydrate, 7 g protein

Diabetic exchanges: 2 vegetable, 1 meat/cheese, 1 milk, ½ fat

Chicken Cheddar Wraps

4 boneless, skinless chicken breast halves (1 pound)
½ cup (4 ounces) fat-free sour cream
¾ cup chunky salsa
2 tablespoons light mayonnaise
1 cup (4 ounces) fat-free shredded cheddar cheese
½ cup thinly sliced fresh mushrooms
2 cups shredded lettuce
6 low-carb, fat-free flour tortillas
Tomato wedges

Cook chicken in skillet coated with nonstick cooking spray. Let cool and dice. Set aside.

In a bowl combine the sour cream, salsa, and mayonnaise. Stir in chicken, cheese, and mushrooms.

Divide lettuce equally on tortillas. Place ½ cup chicken mixture on each tortilla. Fold in half over filling, garnish with tomato, and serve.

Yield: 6 wraps

Nutritional analysis: One wrap equals 167 calories, 3 g fat, 17 g carbohydrate, 18 g protein

Diabetic exchanges: 1½ meat/cheese, 1 starch

Garden Tuna Sandwiches

2 cans (6 ounces) water-packed tuna, drained
½ cup chopped, peeled cucumber
½ shredded carrot
¼ cup finely chopped green onions
½ cup fat-free mayonnaise
¼ cup Dijon mustard

1 tablespoon fat-free sour cream
1 teaspoon lemon juice
¼ teaspoon pepper
8 slices whole-wheat bread
4 lettuce leaves

In a bowl combine the tuna, cucumber, carrot, onions, mayonnaise, mustard, sour cream, lemon juice, and pepper. Spread on four slices of bread. Top with lettuce and remaining bread.

Yield: 4 servings

Nutritional analysis: One sandwich equals 236 calories, 4 g fat, 32 g carbohydrate, 18 g protein

Diabetic exchanges: 1½ meat/cheese, 2 starch, 1 vegetable, ½ fat

Italian Mushroom Salad

2 pounds fresh mushrooms, quartered
3 medium tomatoes, cut into wedges
1 cup fat-free Italian salad dressing
1 teaspoon dried parsley flakes
½ teaspoon garlic powder
¼ cup chopped onion
½ teaspoon dried basil
3 cups fresh spinach leaves
4 turkey bacon strips, cooked and chopped

Place mushrooms and tomatoes in a large shallow dish. Combine the next 5 ingredients and drizzle over mushrooms and tomatoes. Cover and refrigerate overnight, stirring once.

Line a serving platter or bowl with spinach. Using a slotted spoon, arrange vegetables over spinach. Sprinkle with turkey bacon and serve.

Yield: 8 servings

Nutritional analysis: One cup serving equals 37 calories, 1 g fat, 8 g
  carbohydrate, 1 g protein

Diabetic exchanges: 1 vegetable

Mushroom Turkey Burger

2 pounds ground turkey breast
1 can (4 ounces) mushroom stems and pieces, drained
¼ cup egg substitute
½ cup chopped onion
¼ cup ketchup
1 teaspoon Italian seasoning
¼ teaspoon pepper
¼ teaspoon Worcestershire sauce

In a bowl combine all ingredients. Divide into 8 patties and grill, covered, over medium heat until meat is no longer pink, turning once.

Yield: 8 servings

Nutritional analysis: One serving equals 186 calories, 6 g fat, 4 g
  carbohydrate, 29 g protein

Diabetic exchanges: 2 meat/cheese, 1 vegetable, 1 fat

Soft Chicken Tacos

4 boneless skinless chicken breast halves (1 pound), cut into cubes
1 can (15 ounces) black beans, rinsed and drained
1 cup salsa
1 tablespoon taco seasoning
½ cup fat-free sour cream
6 low-carb, fat-free flour tortillas

Optional: Shredded lettuce
Fat-free shredded cheddar cheese
Diced tomatoes
Sliced green onions

In a skillet that has been coated with nonstick cooking spray, cook chicken until juices run clear. Add beans, salsa, and taco seasoning. Heat through. Remove from heat and add sour cream. Spoon the chicken mixture down the center of each tortilla. Garnish with toppings of your choice.

Yield: 6 servings

Nutritional analysis: One taco without vegetables and cheese equals 196 calories, 4 g fat, 18 g carbohydrate, 22 g protein

Diabetic exchanges: 1½ meat/cheese, 1 starch, 1 vegetable, ½ fat

Spinach Chicken Wraps

1 package (10 ounces) fresh spinach
½ cup chopped fresh mushrooms
1 green onion, finely chopped
1 garlic clove, minced
1 tablespoon olive oil
2 egg whites, lightly beaten
¼ cup crumbled feta cheese
¼ cup dry bread crumbs
¼ teaspoon dried rosemary, crushed
4 boneless, skinless chicken breast halves (1 pound)
½ teaspoon dried basil
½ teaspoon dried thyme
¼ teaspoon pepper
4 low-carb, fat-free flour tortillas

In a large saucepan place spinach in a steamer basket over 1 inch of boiling water. Cover and steam for 2 to 3 minutes or until just wilted. When cool enough to handle, squeeze spinach dry and finely chop.

In a nonstick skillet sauté the mushrooms, onion, and garlic in oil until tender. Add spinach. Cook and stir for 2 minutes and then transfer to a bowl. Add egg whites, cheese, and bread crumbs; mix well.

Flatten chicken to ¼-in. thickness. Combine basil, thyme, and pepper and rub over one side of chicken.

Place chicken on tortillas. Spread spinach mixture on chicken and roll up lengthwise. Secure with toothpicks.

In a large saucepan boil 1 inch of water, place wraps in a steamer basket over water, cover and steam for 12 to 15 minutes or until chicken is no longer pink.

Yield: 4 servings

Nutritional analysis: One serving equals 238 calories, 6 g fat, 16 g carbohydrate, 30 g protein

Diabetic exchanges: 2 meat/cheese, 1 vegetable, 1 fat, 1 starch,

Vegetarian Burritos

10 egg whites (or equivalent egg substitute)
¼ teaspoon pepper
1 cup salsa
¼ cup chopped onion
1 cup (4 ounces) fat-free shredded cheddar cheese
8 low-carb, fat-free flour tortillas

In a bowl beat the eggs and pepper together. Pour into a skillet that has been coated with nonstick cooking spray. Cook and stir over medium heat until eggs are partially set. Add salsa and onion. Continue cooking and stir until eggs are completely set. Sprinkle with cheese.

Spoon ½ cup down the center of each tortilla. Fold ends and sides over filling. Serve immediately.

Yield: 8 servings

Nutritional analysis: One serving equals 146 calories, 2 g fat, 20 g carbohydrate, 12 g protein

Diabetic exchanges: 1 meat/cheese, 1 starch, 1 vegetable

Dinner

Blueberry Chicken

4 boneless skinless chicken breast halves (1 pound)
1 tablespoon canola oil
¼ cup apricot preserves or fruit spread
3 tablespoons Dijon mustard
¼ cup white wine vinegar or cider vinegar
1 cup fresh or frozen blueberries

In a large skillet over medium heat, cook chicken in oil for about 5 minutes on each side until lightly browned.

Combine preserves and mustard. Spoon over chicken. Reduce heat to low; cover and simmer for 20 minutes or until chicken juices run clear.

With a slotted spoon, remove chicken and keep warm in a serving dish.

Add vinegar to skillet and bring to a boil. Reduce heat, simmer uncovered for 3 minutes or until sauce is reduced by one-third, stirring occasionally. Stir in blueberries.

Spoon sauce over chicken. Serve with rice if desired.

Yield: 4 servings

Nutritional analysis: One serving (prepared with 100 percent apricot fruit spread; rice not included) equals 206 calories, 6 g fat, 10 g carbohydrate, 28 g protein

Diabetic exchanges: 2 meat/cheese, 1 fruit, 1 fat

Broccoli-Cabbage Slaw

2 cups shredded cabbage
2 cups broccoli florets
1 cup cauliflowerets
1 medium red onion, thinly sliced
¼ cup reduced-fat mayonnaise
¼ cup fat-free plain yogurt
¼ cup reduced-fat sour cream
¼ cup reduced-fat shredded Parmesan cheese

In a salad bowl combine the cabbage, broccoli, cauliflower, and onion.

In a separate small bowl combine the remaining ingredients. Pour over vegetables and toss to coat. Cover and refrigerate until serving.

Yield: 6 servings

Nutritional analysis: A ¾ cup serving equals 116 calories, 6 g fat, 15 g carbohydrate, 5 g protein

Diabetic exchanges: ½ meat/cheese, 1 vegetable, 1 fat

Cajun Salmon Steaks

2 salmon steaks (6 ounces, 1 inch thick)
½ teaspoon Worcestershire sauce
½ teaspoon lemon juice
½ teaspoon Cajun or Creole seasoning
½ cup diced green pepper
½ cup diced red pepper

Place salmon in an ungreased 8-inch square microwave-safe dish. Rub top with Worcestershire sauce and lemon juice. Sprinkle with Cajun seasoning and then put peppers on top. Cover and microwave on high for 5 to 6 minutes or until fish flakes easily with a fork. Turn once while cooking. Let stand covered for 1 minute before serving.

Yield: 2 servings

Nutritional analysis: One serving equals 268 calories, 12 g fat, 4 g
    carbohydrate, 36 g protein

Diabetic exchanges: 2½ meat/cheese, 2 fat, ½ vegetable

Chicken Burritos

¼ cup olive oil
¼ cup lime juice
4 garlic cloves, minced
1 tablespoon minced fresh parsley or 1 teaspoon dried parsley
    flakes
1 teaspoon ground cumin
1 teaspoon dried oregano
¼ teaspoon pepper
4 boneless, skinless chicken breast halves (1 pound)
6 low-carb, fat-free flour tortillas
Shredded lettuce, diced tomatoes, and other vegetables of your
    choice

In a large resealable plastic bag or shallow glass container, combine the first 7 ingredients. Shake or stir well. Add chicken and turn to coat. Seal or cover and refrigerate 8 hours or overnight, turning occasionally. Drain and discard marinade.

Grill chicken uncovered over medium heat for 5 to 7 minutes on each side or until juices run clear. Cut into thin strips. Serve in tortillas or taco shells with vegetables.

Yield: 6 servings

Nutritional analysis: One serving equals 201 calories, 5 g fat, 15 g carbohydrate, 24 g protein, depending on vegetables used

Diabetic exchanges: 2 meat/cheese, 1 startch, ½ fat, ½ vegetable

Chicken Veggie Stew

2 pounds boneless skinless chicken breasts, cubed
1 can (14½ ounces) Italian diced tomatoes, undrained
2 medium potatoes, peeled and cut into ½-inch cubes
6 medium carrots, chopped
4 celery stalks, chopped
1 large onion, chopped
1 medium green pepper, chopped
2 cans (4 ounces *each*) mushrooms, drained
2 low-sodium chicken bouillon cubes
1 teaspoon chili powder
¼ teaspoon pepper
1 tablespoon cornstarch
2 cups water

In a slow cooker combine the first 11 ingredients.

In a small bowl, combine cornstarch and water until smooth.

Stir into chicken mixture.

Cover and cook on low for 8 to 10 hours or until vegetables are tender.

Yield: 8 servings

Nutritional analysis: One serving equals 220 calories, 4 g fat, 16 g carbohydrate, 30 g protein

Diabetic exchanges: 2 meat/cheese, 2 vegetable, ½ startch, ½ fat

Chili Chicken Breasts

1 teaspoon chili powder
½ teaspoon ground cumin
¼ teaspoon garlic powder
¼ teaspoon cayenne pepper
4 boneless, skinless chicken breast halves (1 pound)
1 teaspoon canola oil
¼ cup chopped green onions
1 jalapeno pepper, seeded and finely chopped
1 garlic clove, minced
1 can (14½ ounces) diced tomatoes, undrained
1 teaspoon cornstarch
2 teaspoons water

Combine the first 4 ingredients and rub over chicken.

In a nonstick skillet, brown chicken in oil on both sides. Add onions, jalapeno, and garlic. Sauté for 1 minute. Add tomatoes and bring to a boil. Reduce heat, cover and simmer for 15 to 20 minutes. Remove chicken only and keep warm. Leave rest of ingredients in skillet.

In a small bowl combine cornstarch and water until smooth. Stir into tomato mixture in skillet. Bring to a boil. Cook and stir for 1 minute or until slightly thickened. Serve over chicken.

Yield: 4 servings

Nutritional analysis: One serving equals 164 calories, 4 g fat, 4 g carbohydrate, 28 g protein

Diabetic exchanges: 2 meat/cheese, 1 vegetable, ½ fat

Cilantro Lime Cod

4 cod fillets (2 pounds)
¼ teaspoon pepper

1 tablespoon dried minced onion
1 garlic clove, minced
1 tablespoon olive oil
1 teaspoon ground cumin
¼ cup minced fresh cilantro or parsley
2 limes, thinly sliced
1 tablespoon canola oil-based butter

Place each fillet on a 12 x 15 piece of heavy-duty foil. Sprinkle with pepper.

In a small saucepan sauté onion and garlic in oil. Stir in cumin. Spoon over fillets. Sprinkle with cilantro. Place lime slices over each fillet and drizzle with butter. Fold foil around fish, seal tightly, and place on a baking sheet.

Bake at 375 degrees for 35 to 40 minutes or until fish flakes easily with a fork.

Yield: 8 servings

Nutritional analysis: One serving equals 209 calories, 6 g fat, 3 g carbohydrate, 28 g protein

Diabetic exchanges: 2 meat/cheese, 1 fat

Creamed Mushroom Turkey

1 boneless turkey breast (3 pounds), halved
1 tablespoon canola oil-based butter, melted
2 tablespoons dried parsley flakes
½ teaspoon dried tarragon
½ teaspoon salt
¼ teaspoon pepper
1 jar (4½ ounces) sliced mushrooms, drained or 1 cup sliced fresh mushrooms
½ cup chicken broth

2 tablespoons cornstarch
¼ cup cold water

Place the turkey in a slow cooker. Brush with butter. Sprinkle with parsley, tarragon, salt, and pepper. Top with mushrooms. Pour broth over all.

Cover and cook on low for 7 to 8 hours.

Remove turkey and keep warm.

Skim fat from cooking juices. In a saucepan, combine cornstarch and water until smooth. Gradually add cooking juices. Bring to a boil; cook and stir for 2 minutes or until thickened. Serve over the turkey.

Yield: 12 servings

Nutritional analysis: One serving equals 191 calories, 7 g fat, 4 g carbohydrate, 28 g protein

Diabetic exchanges: 2 meat/cheese, 1 fat, ½ vegetable

Creamy Chicken Enchiladas

1 small onion, chopped
1 can (10¾ ounces) reduced-fat, reduced-sodium condensed cream of chicken soup, undiluted
1 can (10 ounces) diced tomatoes and green chilies, undrained
1 cup (8 ounces) fat-free sour cream
1 cup (4 ounces) shredded fat-free cheddar cheese
1 cup (4 ounces) shredded reduced-fat mozzarella cheese
6 low-carb flour tortillas
3 cooked chicken breasts (cubed)

In a skillet or saucepan coated with nonstick cooking spray, sauté onion until tender. Remove from heat. Add soup, tomatoes, sour cream, ¾ cup cheddar cheese, and ¾ cup mozzarella cheese. Mix well.

Divide evenly on each tortilla, top with ½ of a cubed chicken breast. Roll up tightly.

Place seam side down in a 9 x 13 baking dish coated with nonstick cooking spray. Top with remaining soup mixture; sprinkle with remaining cheeses. Bake uncovered at 350 degrees for 20 to 25 minutes or until heated through.

Yield: 6 servings

Nutritional analysis: One serving equals 226 calories, 6 g fat, 21 g carbohydrate, 22 g protein

Diabetic exchanges: 1½ meat/cheese, 1 vegetable, 1 starch, 1 fat

Creamy Pea Salad

2 medium carrots, chopped
1 package (16 ounces) frozen peas
1 celery rib, thinly sliced
¼ cup cubed, reduced-fat mozzarella cheese
2 green onions, thinly sliced
2 tablespoons buttermilk
2 tablespoons plain nonfat yogurt
1 teaspoon fat-free mayonnaise
½ teaspoon cider or red wine vinegar
½ teaspoon dried basil
¼ teaspoon pepper

In a saucepan cook carrots in a small amount of boiling water for 2 minutes. Add peas and cook 5 more minutes. Drain. Rinse in cold water and drain again. Place in a bowl and add celery, cheese, and onions.

In a separate bowl combine remaining ingredients and pour over pea mixture. Toss to coat. Cover and refrigerate for at least 1 hour.

Yield: 5 servings

Nutritional analysis: One ¾-cup serving equals 103 calories, 3 g fat, 15 g carbohydrate, 4 g protein

Diabetic exchanges: 1 vegetable, ½ starch, ½ fat

Curry Chicken Breasts

4 boneless skinless chicken breast halves (4 ounces each)
1 tablespoon canola oil
¼ cup Worcestershire sauce
2 tablespoons chili sauce
2 teaspoons curry powder
1 teaspoon garlic powder
¼ teaspoon hot pepper sauce
¼ cup chopped onion

In a large skillet, brown chicken on both sides in oil.

In a bowl, combine the Worcestershire sauce, chili sauce, curry powder, garlic powder, and hot pepper sauce. Pour over chicken. Add onion. Reduce heat. Cover and simmer for 9 to 11 minutes.

Yield: 4 servings

Nutritional analysis: One serving equals 186 calories, 6 g fat, 4 g carbohydrate, 28 g protein

Diabetic exchanges: 2 meat/cheese, 1 fat

Dill Salmon

1 salmon fillet (1 pound)
1½ teaspoons dill weed
½ cup fat-free plain yogurt
½ teaspoon brown sugar
½ teaspoon salt-free seasoning blend

Place the salmon in a 9 x 13 baking dish coated with nonstick cooking spray. Sprinkle salmon with ½ teaspoon dill.

Cover and bake at 375 degrees for 20 to 25 minutes or until the fish flakes easily with a fork.

In a small saucepan combine the yogurt, brown sugar, seasoning blend, and remaining dill. Cook and stir over low heat until heated through.

Place salmon on a serving dish and cover with sauce.

Yield: 4 servings

Nutritional analysis: One serving equals 227 calories, 12 g fat, 3 g carbohydrate, 24 g protein

Diabetic exchanges: 2 meat/cheese, 2 fat

Garlic Chicken

½ cup dry bread crumbs
¼ cup reduced-fat grated Parmesan cheese
2 tablespoons minced fresh parsley
¼ teaspoon pepper
¼ cup skim milk
6 boneless, skinless chicken breast halves (1½ pounds)
¼ cup canola oil-based butter
2 garlic cloves, minced
2 tablespoons lemon juice
Pinch of paprika

In a large resealable plastic bag, combine the first 4 ingredients. Place milk in a shallow bowl. Dip chicken in milk and then place in bag. Shake. Place in a greased 9 x 13 baking dish.

Combine the butter, garlic, and lemon juice. Drizzle over the chicken. Sprinkle with paprika.

Bake uncovered at 350 degrees for 25 to 30 minutes.

Yield: 6 servings

Nutritional analysis: One serving equals 172 calories, 6 g fat, 4 g carbohydrate, 30 g protein

Diabetic exchanges: 2 meat/cheese, 1 fat

Herbed Lime Chicken

1 bottle (16 ounces) fat-free Italian salad dressing
½ cup lime juice
1 lime, halved and sliced
3 garlic cloves, minced
1 teaspoon dried thyme
8 boneless, skinless chicken breast halves (2 pounds)

In a bowl combine the first 5 ingredients. Put ½ cup of mixture in covered container and refrigerate. Pour remaining mixture into a large resealable plastic bag. Add chicken, seal bag, and turn to coat. Refrigerate for 8 to 10 hours. Drain and discard marinade.

Grill chicken uncovered over medium heat for 5 minutes. Turn chicken and baste with the ½ cup reserved marinade. Grill 5 to 7 more minutes, basting occasionally.

Yield: 8 servings

Nutritional analysis: One serving equals 172 calories, 4 g fat, 6 g carbohydrate, 28 g protein

Diabetic exchanges: 2 meat/cheese, ½ fat

Italian Chicken Cutlets

6 boneless skinless chicken breast halves (1½ pounds)
1 cup dry bread crumbs
½ cup nonfat Parmesan cheese topping
2 tablespoons wheat germ
1 teaspoon dried basil

½ teaspoon garlic powder
1 cup plain fat-free yogurt
Refrigerated butter-flavored spray

Flatten chicken to ½-inch thickness.

In a shallow dish combine the bread crumbs, Parmesan topping, wheat germ, basil, and garlic powder.

Place yogurt in separate shallow dish.

Dip chicken into yogurt and coat with crumb mixture.

Place in a 10 x 15 baking pan coated with nonstick cooking spray. Spritz chicken with butter-flavored spray.

Bake uncovered at 350 degrees for 20 to 25 minutes or until the juices run clear.

Yield: 6 servings

Nutritional analysis: One serving equals 270 calories, 5 g fat, 15 g carbohydrate, 32 g protein

Diabetic exchanges: 2 meat/cheese, 1 starch, ½ fat

Italian Orange Roughy Fillets

1 pound orange roughy fillets
½ cup tomato juice
1 tablespoon white vinegar
1 envelope Italian salad dressing mix
¼ cup chopped green onions
¼ cup chopped green pepper

Place fish fillets in a shallow 2-quart glass baking dish, positioning the thickest portion of fish toward the outside edges.

Combine tomato juice, vinegar, and salad dressing mix. Pour over fish, making sure some sauce gets under the fish.

Cover and refrigerate for 30 minutes.

Sprinkle fish and sauce with green onions and green pepper.

Cover and bake at 400 for 15 minutes or until fish flakes easily with fork. Let stand covered for 2 minutes before serving.

Yield: 4 servings

Nutritional analysis: One serving equals 122 calories, 2 g fat, 5 g carbohydrate, 21 g protein

Diabetic exchanges: 1 meat/cheese, ½ vegetable

Italian-Tomato Chicken

4 boneless, skinless chicken breast halves (1 pound)
½ cup fat-free Italian salad dressing
8 tomato slices, ¼-inch thick
4 teaspoons seasoned bread crumbs
1 teaspoon minced fresh basil or ¼ teaspoon dried basil
1 tablespoon grated, reduced-fat Parmesan cheese

Place chicken in a shallow bowl. Pour ¼ cup Italian dressing over chicken. Cover and refrigerate for 2 hours. Transfer chicken to a shallow baking dish. Discard marinade.

Drizzle chicken with remaining dressing. Cover and bake at 400 degrees for 10 minutes.

Top each chicken breast with tomato slices, crumbs, basil, and cheese. Cover and bake for 10 minutes. Uncover and bake 10 to 15 minutes or until chicken juices run clear.

Yield: 4 servings

Nutritional analysis: One serving equals 164 calories, 4 g fat, 8 g carbohydrate, 28 g protein

Diabetic exchanges: 1½ meat/cheese, ½ vegetable, ½ fat

Lean and Meaty Spaghetti Sauce

1½ pounds ground turkey breast
½ pound bulk Italian sausage
1 medium green pepper, chopped
1 medium onion, chopped
8 garlic cloves, minced
3 cans (14½ ounces *each*) diced tomatoes, drained
2 cans (15 ounces *each*) tomato sauce
2 cans (6 ounces *each*) tomato paste
¼ cup sugar
2 tablespoons Italian seasoning
1 tablespoon dried basil
1 teaspoon salt
½ teaspoon pepper
Hot cooked spaghetti

In a large skillet over medium heat, cook turkey and sausage until no longer pink. Drain and transfer to a 5-quart slow cooker. Stir in green pepper, onion, garlic, tomatoes, tomato sauce, tomato paste, sugar, and various seasonings. Mix well. Cover and cook on low for 8 hours or until bubbly. Serve over hot spaghetti.

Yield: 12 servings

Nutritional analysis: One serving (calculated without spaghetti) equals 180 calories, 4 g fat, 12 g carbohydrate, 24 g protein

Diabetic exchanges: 1½ meat/cheese, 1 starch, 1 vegetable

Lean Swedish Meatballs

2 egg whites, lightly beaten
¼ cup ketchup
¾ cup dry bread crumbs
2 tablespoons dried parsley flakes

2 tablespoons Worcestershire sauce
1 teaspoon onion powder
1 teaspoon garlic powder
1 teaspoon pepper
½ teaspoon salt
½ teaspoon chili powder
3 pounds ground turkey breast
2 envelopes brown gravy mix
½ cup fat-free sour cream

In a bowl, combine the first 10 ingredients. Crumble meat over mixture and mix well. Shape into 1-inch balls (about 6 dozen).

In a bowl combine brown gravy mix and water according to package instructions.

Place meatballs in a single layer in ungreased 10x15 baking pans. Coat with gravy mix. Bake at 400 degrees for 20 minutes or until meat is no longer pink, turning often. Remove from the oven. Stir in sour cream. Let cool.

Yield: 75 meatballs per batch, 15 servings

Nutritional analysis: Five Swedish meatballs equal 223 calories, 7 g fat, 8 g carbohydrate, 32 g protein

Diabetic exchanges: 2 meat/cheese, ½ starch, 1 fat

Lemon Baked Salmon

1 salmon fillet (2 pounds)
2 tablespoons canola oil-based butter
¼ cup white wine
2 tablespoons lemon juice
½ teaspoon pepper
½ teaspoon dried tarragon
Sliced lemon

Pat salmon dry. Place in a 9 x 13 baking dish coated with nonstick cooking spray. Brush with butter.

Combine wine, lemon juice, pepper, and tarragon. Pour over salmon. Top with lemon slices.

Bake uncovered at 425 degrees for 20 to 25 minutes or until fish flakes easily with a fork.

Yield: 8 servings

Nutritional analysis: A 4-ounce serving equals 192 calories, 8 g fat, 2 g carbohydrate, 28 g protein

Diabetic exchanges: 1½ meat/cheese, 1 fat

Lemon Chicken

½ cup water
¼ cup lemon juice
2 tablespoons dried minced onion
1 tablespoon dried parsley flakes
1 tablespoon Worcestershire sauce
1 garlic clove, minced
1 teaspoon dill weed
½ teaspoon curry powder
½ teaspoon pepper
8 boneless, skinless chicken breast halves (2 pounds), cut up

In a large resealable bag or shallow glass container, combine the first 9 ingredients. Add chicken, turning to coat. Seal or cover and refrigerate for 4 to 6 hours. Drain and discard marinade.

Grill chicken, covered, over low heat for 50 to 60 minutes or until juices run clear, turning several times.

Yield: 8 servings

Nutritional analysis: One serving equals 156 calories, 4 g fat, 2 g carbohydrates, 28 g protein

Diabetic exchanges: 1½ meat/cheese, ½ fat

Lemon Fish

1 pound whitefish or sole fillets
¼ cup lemon juice
1 teaspoon olive oil
2 teaspoons salt-free lemon-pepper seasoning
1 small onion, thinly sliced
1 teaspoon dried parsley flakes

Cut fish into serving-size pieces. Place in an ungreased 7 x 11 baking dish. Drizzle with lemon juice and oil. Sprinkle on lemon pepper. Arrange onion over fish and sprinkle with parsley. Cover and let stand for 5 minutes.

Bake at 350 degrees for 20 minutes or until fish flakes easily with a fork.

Yield: 4 servings

Nutritional analysis: One serving equals 156 calories, 6 g fat, 2 g carbohydrate, 28 g protein

Diabetic exchanges: 1½ meat/cheese, 1 fat

Light Spinach Quiche

3 ounces fat-free cream cheese
1 cup skim milk
8 egg whites
¼ teaspoon pepper
3 cups (12 ounces) shredded fat-free cheddar cheese

1 package (10 ounces) frozen chopped spinach, thawed and squeezed
    dry
1 cup frozen chopped broccoli, thawed and well-drained
1 small onion, finely chopped
5 fresh mushrooms, sliced

In a small mixing bowl, beat cream cheese. Add milk, egg whites, and pepper. Beat until smooth. Stir in remaining ingredients. Transfer to a 10-inch quiche pan coated with nonstick cooking spray.

Bake at 350 degrees for 45 to 50 minutes or until a knife inserted near the center comes out clean.

Yield: 8 servings

Nutritional analysis: One serving equals 122 calories, 2 g fat, 8 g
    carbohydrate, 18 g protein

Diabetic exchanges: 1 meat/cheese, 1 vegetable, 1 milk

Light Turkey Salad Tortillas

12 ounces cooked turkey, shredded or cubed
1 cup (4 ounces) fat-free shredded cheddar cheese
¾ cup finely chopped celery
½ cup finely chopped onion
1 can (2¼ ounces) sliced olives, drained
½ cup light mayonnaise
¼ cup picante sauce
6 low-carb flour tortillas (7 inches)

In a bowl, combine the first 7 ingredients and mix well. Evenly divide filling of center on each tortilla. Fold sides and ends over filling and roll up.

Place in a shallow, microwave-safe dish. Cover and microwave on high for 2 to 3 minutes or until cheese is melted and filling is hot.

Yield: 6 servings

Nutritional analysis: One serving equals 151 calories, 3 g fat, 16 g carbohydrate, 15 g protein

Diabetic exchanges: 1 meat/cheese, 1 starch, 1 vegetable, ½ fat

Mini Turkey Loaves

4 egg whites
½ cup fat-free plain yogurt
1 can (6 ounces) tomato paste
2 tablespoons Worcestershire sauce
½ cup quick-cooking oats
1 small onion, chopped
2 tablespoons dried parsley flakes
1 teaspoon salt
½ teaspoon garlic powder
½ teaspoon pepper
2 pounds ground turkey breast
½ cup low-carb ketchup

In a large bowl combine the first 10 ingredients. Crumble turkey over mixture and mix well. Shape into 8 loaves. Place on a rack coated with nonstick cooking spray in a shallow baking pan.

Bake uncovered at 350 degrees for 30 minutes. Spoon ketchup over the loaves. Bake 15 minutes longer.

Yield: 8 servings

Nutritional analysis: One serving equals 172 calories, 4 g fat, 2 g carbohydrates, 30 g protein

Diabetic exchanges: 2 meat/cheese, ½ fat, ½ vegetable

Mushroom Spinach Tart

2 tablespoons seasoned bread crumbs
½ pound fresh mushrooms, sliced
½ cup chopped onion
1 tablespoon olive oil
1 package (10 ounces) frozen chopped spinach, thawed and
    squeezed dry
1 cup skim milk
1 cup egg substitute
¼ teaspoon salt
¼ teaspoon pepper
1 cup shredded reduced-fat Mexican cheese
½ cup grated reduced-fat Parmesan cheese

Coat a 9-inch pie plate with nonstick cooking spray. Sprinkle bottom and sides with bread crumbs, shaking out excess. Set plate aside.

In a nonstick skillet sauté mushrooms and onion in oil for 12 to 14 minutes or until all of the liquid has evaporated. Remove from heat and stir in spinach.

In a bowl combine the milk, egg substitute, salt, and pepper. Stir in the spinach mixture, 1 cup Mexican cheese blend, and Parmesan cheese. Pour into pie plate.

Bake at 350 degrees for 35 to 40 minutes or until a knife inserted near the center comes out clean.

Let stand for 5 minutes before slicing.

Yield: 8 servings

Nutritional analysis: One piece equals 176 calories, 8 g fat, 10 g carbohydrate, 16 g protein

Diabetic exchanges: 1 meat/cheese, 1 milk, 1 vegetable, 1 fat, ½ starch

Orange Roughy Primavera

1 tablespoon canola oil-based butter
4 orange roughy fillets (4 ounces each), thawed
2 tablespoons lemon juice
Pinch of pepper
1 garlic clove, minced
1 tablespoon olive oil
1 cup broccoli florets
1 cup cauliflowerets
1 cup julienned carrots
1 cup sliced fresh mushrooms
½ cup sliced celery
¼ teaspoon dried basil
¼ teaspoon salt
¼ cup reduced-fat, grated Parmesan cheese

Spread butter in a 9 x 13 baking dish. Lightly coat fish with butter and place in pan. Sprinkle with lemon juice and pepper.

Bake uncovered at 450 degrees for 5 minutes.

In a large skillet over medium heat sauté garlic in oil. Add the next 7 ingredients. Stir-fry until vegetables are crisp-tender (2 to 3 minutes). Spoon over the fish and sprinkle with cheese.

Bake uncovered at 450 degrees for 3 to 5 minutes or until fish flakes easily with a fork.

Yield: 4 servings

Nutritional analysis: One serving equals 215 calories, 7 g fat, 10 g carbohydrate, 28 g protein

Diabetic exchanges: 2 meat/cheese, 1½ vegetable, 1 fat

Oriental Sesame Chicken

1 pound boneless skinless chicken breasts, cubed
1 tablespoon canola oil
¼ cup light soy sauce
¼ cup sesame seeds
1 large onion, sliced
2 jars (4½ ounces *each*) sliced mushrooms, drained, or 2 cups sliced
    fresh mushrooms

In a large skillet cook chicken in oil until no longer pink. Stir in soy sauce and sesame seeds. Cook and stir over medium heat for 5 minutes. Remove chicken with a slotted spoon; set aside and keep warm.

In the same skillet, sauté onion and mushrooms until onion is tender.

Return chicken to pan and heat through.

Yield: 4 servings

Nutritional analysis: One serving equals 212 calories, 8 g fat, 6 g
    carbohydrate, 29 g protein

Diabetic exchanges: 2 meat/cheese, 1 fat, 1 vegetable

Parmesan Chicken

½ cup dry bread crumbs
½ cup grated reduced-fat Parmesan cheese
2 tablespoons minced fresh parsley
1 garlic clove, minced
¼ teaspoon pepper
4 egg whites
8 boneless, skinless chicken breast halves (2 pounds)
½ cup sliced almonds
Butter-flavored cooking spray

In a shallow bowl combine the first 5 ingredients.

In another shallow bowl beat the egg whites. Dip chicken in egg whites and then coat with crumb mixture.

Place in a 9 x 13 baking dish coated with nonstick cooking spray. Sprinkle almonds over chicken. Spritz lightly with butter-flavored cooking spray. Bake uncovered at 350 degrees for 30 minutes.

Yield: 8 servings

Nutritional analysis: One serving equals 216 calories, 8 g fat, 6 g carbohydrate, 30 g protein

Diabetic exchanges: 2 meat/cheese, 1 fat, ½ starch

Southwest Chicken

4 boneless skinless chicken breast halves (1 pound)
16 ounces picante sauce
2 tablespoons brown sugar
1 tablespoon mustard

Spray shallow 2 quart baking dish with nonstick cooking spray and put chicken in. In a small bowl, combine the picante sauce, brown sugar, and mustard. Pour over chicken.

Bake uncovered at 400 degrees for 30 to 35 minutes. Serve over rice if desired.

Yield: 4 servings

Nutritional analysis: One serving (calculated without rice) equals 224 calories, 4 g fat, 19 g carbohydrate, 28 g protein

Diabetic exchanges: 2 meat/cheese, 1 starch, ½ fat

Spicy Haddock

2 pounds haddock fillets, thawed
1 can (4 ounces) chopped green chilies

1 tablespoon canola oil
1 tablespoon soy sauce
2 tablespoons Worcestershire sauce
1 teaspoon paprika
½ teaspoon garlic powder
½ teaspoon chili powder
Dash of hot pepper sauce

Place fillets in a 9 x 13 baking dish that has been coated with non-stick cooking spray.

Combine remaining ingredients and spoon over fish.

Bake uncovered at 350 degrees for 20 to 25 minutes or until fish flakes easily with a fork.

Yield: 8 servings

Nutritional analysis: One 4-ounce serving equals 155 calories, 5 g fat, 2 g carbohydrate, 28 g protein

Diabetic exchanges: 2 meat/cheese, ½ fat, ½ vegetable

Spicy White Chili

2 pounds boneless skinless chicken breasts, cubed
1 small onion, chopped
2 cups low-sodium chicken broth
1 can (4 ounces) chopped green chilies
½ teaspoon garlic powder
½ teaspoon dried oregano
½ teaspoon minced fresh cilantro or parsley
¼ teaspoon cayenne pepper
1 can (15 ounces) white kidney or cannelini beans, rinsed and
    drained

In a saucepan coated with nonstick cooking spray, sauté chicken and onion until juices run clear; drain if desired. Stir in broth, chilies, garlic powder, oregano, cilantro, and cayenne. Bring to a boil. Reduce heat; simmer uncovered, for 30 minutes. Stir in beans and cook for 10 minutes.

Yield: 8 servings

Nutritional analysis: One serving equals 220 calories, 4 g fat, 14 g
   carbohydrate, 32 g protein

Diabetic exchanges: 2½ meat/cheese, ½ fat, 1 vegetable, ½ starch

Stuffed Sole

2 tablespoons canola oil-based butter
2 tablespoons lemon juice
½ teaspoon salt
¼ teaspoon pepper
1 package (10 ounces) frozen, chopped broccoli, thawed and
   drained
1 cup cooked rice
1 cup (4 ounces) shredded reduced-fat cheddar cheese
8 sole or whitefish fillets (4 ounces each)
Paprika

In a small bowl combine the butter, lemon juice, salt, and pepper.

In another bowl combine the broccoli, rice, cheese, and half of the other mixture. Spoon ½ cup onto each raw fillet.

Roll up fillets and place seam side down in a baking dish coated with nonstick cooking spray. Pour remaining mixture over roll-ups.

Bake uncovered at 350 degrees for 25 minutes or until fish flakes easily with a fork.

Baste with pan drippings, sprinkle with paprika, and serve.

Yield: 8 servings

Nutritional analysis: One serving equals 231 calories, 7 g fat, 12 g
  carbohydrate, 30 g protein

Diabetic exchanges: 2 meat/cheese, 1 fat, 1 vegetable, 1 starch

Sweet and Spicy Chicken

1 pound boneless, skinless chicken breasts, cut into ½-inch cubes
3 tablespoons taco seasoning
1 tablespoon canola oil
1 jar (11 ounces) chunky salsa
½ cup sugar-free peach preserves

Coat chicken with taco seasoning. In a skillet, brown chicken in oil.

Combine salsa and preserves and stir into skillet. Bring to a boil.
Reduce heat. Cover and simmer for 2 to 3 minutes. Serve over rice
if desired.

Yield: 4 servings

Nutritional analysis: One serving without rice equals 197 calories, 5
  g fat, 10 g carbohydrate, 28 g protein

Diabetic exchanges: 2 meat/cheese, 1 fruit, ½ vegetable, ½ fat

Turkey Tortilla Pie

1 teaspoon olive oil
1 small onion, finely chopped
½ teaspoon garlic powder
1 pound ground turkey breast
2 teaspoons chili powder
1 teaspoon dried oregano
½ teaspoon ground cumin
½ teaspoon cayenne pepper
1 can (15 ounces) black beans, rinsed and drained
1 jar (16 ounces) salsa

¾ cup low-sodium chicken broth
8 low-carb, fat-free flour tortillas
½ cup shredded reduced-fat Monterey Jack cheese
¼ cup light sour cream

In a skillet, sauté in oil onion mixed with garlic powder until onion is tender. Add turkey, chili powder, oregano, cumin, and cayenne. Cook and stir over medium heat until turkey is no longer pink.

Stir in beans and remove from heat.

Combine salsa and broth and spread a thin layer on the bottom of a 2½-quart baking dish coated with nonstick cooking spray. Set aside remaining mixture.

Cut tortillas into 1-inch strips and then into thirds. Arrange half over salsa mixture in pan. Top with half the turkey mixture and half of the remaining salsa mixture. Repeat layers. Sprinkle with cheese.

Cover and bake at 350 degrees for 25 minutes or until bubbly.

Before serving top with sour cream.

Yield: 8 servings

Nutritional analysis: One cup serving equals 270 calories, 6 g fat, 32 g carbohydrate, 22 g protein

Diabetic exchanges: 1½ meat/cheese, 2 starch, 1 fat

Zesty Cod

1½ cups water
1 tablespoon lemon juice
2 pounds cod fillets
¼ teaspoon pepper
1 small onion, finely chopped
2 large tomatoes, sliced
½ cup chopped green pepper

½ cup seasoned bread crumbs
¼ cup grated, reduced-fat Parmesan cheese
½ teaspoon dried basil
1 tablespoon olive oil

In a bowl combine the water and lemon juice. Add fish and let sit for 5 minutes. Drain and place in a 7 x 11 baking dish coated with nonstick cooking spray. Sprinkle with pepper. Layer on onion, to-matoes, and green pepper.

Combine the remaining ingredients and sprinkle over top.

Bake uncovered at 375 degrees for 20 to 30 minutes or until fish flakes easily with a fork.

Yield: 8 servings

Nutritional analysis: One serving equals 188 calories, 4 g fat, 10 g carbohydrate, 28 g protein

Diabetic exchanges: 2 meat/cheese, ½ fat, 1 vegetable

Dessert

Blueberry Pie

¼ cup sugar
Sugar substitute, such as Splenda or Stevia, equivalent to
    ¼ cup sugar
2 tablespoons cornstarch
¾ cup water
4 cups fresh or frozen blueberries, thawed
1 premade, reduced-fat graham cracker crust (9 inches)
Fat-free whipped topping

In a saucepan combine sugar, sugar substitute, and cornstarch. Stir in water until smooth. Bring to a boil over medium heat. Cook and stir for 2 minutes. Add blueberries. Cook for 3 minutes, stirring occasionally. Pour into crust. Chill. Garnish with whipped topping and serve.

Yield: 8 servings

Nutritional analysis: One piece equals 94 calories, 2 g fat, 17 g carbohydrate, 2 g protein

Diabetic exchanges: 1 starch, 1 fruit

Cherry Cream Pie

4 ounces fat-free cream cheese, softened
1½ cups sugar-free cherry pie filling
2 cups fat-free whipped topping
1 premade, reduced-fat graham cracker crust (9 inches)

In a mixing bowl beat cream cheese until smooth. Fold in pie filling and whipped topping until blended. Spoon into crust. Cover and freeze for 8 hours or overnight. Remove from freezer 15 minutes before serving.

Yield: 8 servings

Nutritional analysis: One piece equals 94 calories, 2 g fat, 15 g carbohydrate, 4 g protein

Diabetic exchanges: 1 starch, ½ fruit

Chocolate Mousse

¾ cup skim milk
1 package (1.4 ounces) sugar-free instant chocolate pudding mix
½ cup fat-free sour cream
3 ounces fat-free cream cheese, cubed
½ teaspoon vanilla extract
1 carton (8 ounces) fat-free whipped topping

1 tablespoon chocolate cookie crumbs

In a bowl whisk milk and pudding mix for 2 minutes (mixture will be very thick).

In a separate mixing bowl beat the sour cream, cream cheese, and vanilla. Add pudding and mix well. Fold in whipped topping. Spoon into individual dishes. Sprinkle with cookie crumbs. Refrigerate until serving.

Yield: 6 servings

Nutritional analysis: One serving equals 106 calories, 2 g fat, 18 g carbohydrate, 4 g protein

Diabetic exchanges: 1½ starch, ½ milk

Creamy Raspberry Pie

1 package (3 ounces) sugar-free raspberry gelatin
½ cup boiling water
1 cup fat-free frozen vanilla yogurt
1 cup fresh or frozen unsweetened raspberries
¼ cup lime juice
2 cups fat-free whipped topping
1 premade, reduced-fat graham cracker crust (9 inches)
Lime slices and additional raspberries and whipped topping

In a bowl dissolve the gelatin in boiling water. Stir in frozen yogurt until melted. Add raspberries and lime juice. Fold in whipped topping. Spoon into crust. Refrigerate for 3 hours or until firm.

Garnish with lime, raspberries, and whipped topping.

Yield: 8 servings

Nutritional analysis: One slice equals 86 calories, 2 g fat, 13 g carbohydrate, 4 g protein

Diabetic exchanges: 1 starch, ½ fruit

Eggnog Pudding

2 cups skim milk
1 package (3.4 ounces) sugar-free instant vanilla pudding mix
½ teaspoon ground nutmeg
¼ teaspoon rum extract
Additional nutmeg

In a bowl combine the first 4 ingredients. Beat for 2 minutes. Spoon into individual dishes. Chill. Sprinkle with nutmeg and serve.

Yield: 4 servings

Nutritional analysis: One-half cup serving equals 101 calories, 1 g fat, 16 g carbohydrate, 7 g protein.

Diabetic exchanges: 1 starch, 1 milk

Lemon Blueberry Cheesecake

1 package (3 ounces) sugar-free lemon gelatin
1 cup boiling water
2 tablespoons canola oil-based butter
1 tablespoon canola oil
1 cup reduced-fat graham cracker crumbs (about 16 squares)
1 carton (24 ounces) fat-free cottage cheese
¼ cup sugar
Sugar substitute equivalent to ¼ cup sugar

Topping
Sugar substitute equivalent to 2 tablespoons sugar
1½ teaspoons cornstarch
¼ cup water
1½ cups fresh or frozen blueberries
1 teaspoon lemon juice

In a bowl dissolve gelatin in boiling water and let cool.

In a separate bowl combine butter and oil. Add crumbs and blend well. Press onto the bottom of a 9-inch springform pan. Chill.

In a blender process cottage cheese, sugar, and sugar substitute until smooth. While processing, slowly add cooled gelatin. Pour into crust and chill overnight.

For topping, combine sugar substitute and cornstarch in a saucepan. Stir in water until smooth. Add 1 cup blueberries. Bring to a boil. Cook and stir for 2 minutes or until thickened. Stir in lemon juice and cool slightly. Put mixture into blender and process until smooth. Pour into bowl, cover, refrigerate until completely cooled.

The next day carefully run a knife around edge of springform pan to loosen cheesecake and then remove sides of pan. Spread the blueberry mixture over the top. Garnish with remaining blueberries.

Yield: 12 servings

Nutritional analysis: One piece equals 156 calories, 4 g fat, 22 g carbohydrate, 8 g protein

Diabetic exchanges: 1½ starch, ½ fruit, ½ fat, ½ meat/cheese

Lemon Mousse

¼ cup sugar
Sugar substitute, such as Splenda or stevia, equivalent to
     ½ cup sugar
½ cup cornstarch
3 cups skim milk
²/₃ cup lemon juice
1½ teaspoons grated lemon peel
¼ teaspoon vanilla extract
2 cups fat-free whipped topping

In a saucepan combine the sugar, sugar substitute, and cornstarch. Gradually stir in milk until smooth. Bring to a boil over medium heat, stirring constantly. Cook and stir for 2 minutes or until thickened and bubbly. Remove from heat. Stir in lemon juice, peel, and vanilla. Set saucepan in ice. Stir about 5 minutes, until mixture reaches room temperature. Fold in whipped topping. Spoon into dessert dishes. Refrigerate for at least 1 hour before serving.

Yield: 10 servings

Nutritional analysis: One-half cup serving equals 61 calories, 1 g fat, 10 g carbohydrate, 3 g protein

Diabetic exchanges: 1 starch, 1 fruit, ½ milk

Light Carrot Cake

Sugar substitute equivalent to ¼ cup sugar
1 tablespoon canola oil
½ cup sugar-free apple sauce
1/3 cup orange juice concentrate
3 egg whites
1 cup all-purpose flour
1 teaspoon baking powder
1 teaspoon ground cinnamon
½ teaspoon ground allspice
¼ teaspoon baking soda
1 cup grated carrots
2 teaspoons confectioners' sugar

In a mixing bowl combine the first 5 ingredients and beat for 30 seconds. In a separate bowl combine flour, baking powder, cinnamon, allspice, and baking soda. Add to the orange juice mixture and stir well. Add carrots.

Pour into an 8-inch square baking pan that has been coated with nonstick cooking spray. Bake at 350 degrees for 30 minutes or until a toothpick inserted near the center comes out clean.

Let cool, dust with confectioners' sugar, and serve.

Yield: 9 servings

Nutritional analysis: One serving equals 147 calories, 3 g fat, 27 g
  carbohydrate, 3 g protein

Diabetic exchanges: 2 starch, ½ fat, ½ fruit

No-Bake Chocolate Cheesecake

¾ cup reduced-fat graham cracker crumbs (about 12 squares)
2 tablespoons canola oil-based butter
1 envelope unflavored gelatin
1 cup cold water
4 squares (1 ounce *each*) semisweet chocolate, coarsely chopped
4 packages (8 ounces *each*) fat-free cream cheese
Sugar substitute equivalent to 1 cup sugar
¼ cup sugar
¼ cup baking cocoa
2 teaspoons vanilla extract

Topping
2 cups fresh raspberries
1 ounce white candy coating

In a bowl combine cracker crumbs and butter. Press onto the bottom
of a 9-inch springform pan. Bake at 375 degrees for 8 to 10 minutes
or until lightly brown. Cool on a wire rack.

In a small saucepan sprinkle gelatin over cold water and let stand for
1 minute. Heat over low heat, stirring until gelatin is completely dis-
solved. Add the semisweet chocolate and stir until melted.

In a mixing bowl beat the cream cheese, sugar substitute, and sugar
until smooth. Gradually add the chocolate mixture and cocoa. Beat in
vanilla. Pour into crust and refrigerate for 2 to 3 hours or until firm.

Remove cheesecake from refrigerator and arrange raspberries on top.

In a heavy saucepan or microwave, melt white candy coating. Stir until smooth. Drizzle or pipe over berries.

Carefully run a knife around edge of springform pan to loosen and remove sides of pan.

Yield: 12 servings

Nutritional analysis: One slice equals 158 calories, 6 g fat, 27 g carbohydrate, 9 g protein

Diabetic exchanges: 2 starch, 1 meat/cheese, 1 fat

Orange Whip

1 can (11 ounces) mandarin oranges, drained
1 cup (8 ounces) fat-free, low-carb vanilla yogurt
2 tablespoons orange juice concentrate
2 cups fat-free whipped topping

In a bowl combine the oranges, yogurt, and orange juice concentrate. Fold in the whipped topping. Spoon into serving dishes. Cover and freeze until firm. Remove from the freezer 20 minutes before serving.

Yield: 4 servings

Nutritional analysis: Three-quarters cup serving equals 81 calories, 1 g fat, 15 g carbohydrate, 3 g protein

Diabetic exchanges: 1 fruit, 1 starch, ½ milk

Peanut Butter Pudding

2 cups skim milk
4 tablespoons reduced-fat creamy peanut butter
1 package (1 ounce) sugar-free instant vanilla pudding mix

½ cup fat-free whipped topping
4 teaspoons chocolate syrup

In a bowl whisk the milk and peanut butter until blended. Add pudding mix. Whisk for 2 minutes or until slightly thickened. Spoon into dessert dishes. Refrigerate for at least 5 minutes or until set.

Just before serving dollop with whipped topping and drizzle with chocolate syrup.

Yield: 4 servings

Nutritional analysis: One serving equals 172 calories, 8 g fat, 17 g carbohydrate, 8 g protein

Diabetic exchanges: 1 starch, 1 meat/cheese, 1 fat, ½ milk

Pear Squares

1½ pounds pears, sliced
3 tablespoon all-purpose flour
¼ cup unsweetened apple juice concentrate
¾ cup reduced-fat graham cracker crumbs (about 10 squares)
½ teaspoon ground cinnamon
Dash of ground nutmeg
2 tablespoons canola oil-based stick butter
½ cup fat-free whipped topping
Additional ground cinnamon

In a bowl toss the pears, 1 tablespoon of flour, and apple juice concentrate. Spoon into an 8-inch square baking dish coated with nonstick cooking spray.

In a bowl combine the graham cracker crumbs, cinnamon, nutmeg, and 2 tablespoons of flour. Cut in butter until mixture resembles coarse crumbs. Sprinkle over pears.

Bake at 375 degrees for 30 minutes or until pears are tender and topping is lightly browned.

Serve warm or chilled.

Cut into squares and top with whipped topping and cinnamon.

Yield: 9 servings

Nutritional analysis: One serving equals 128 calories, 4 g fat, 22 g carbohydrate, 1 g protein

Diabetic exchanges: 1 starch, 1 fruit, ½ fat

Pumpkin Spice Dip

1 package (8 ounces) fat-free cream cheese
½ cup canned pumpkin
Sugar substitute equivalent to ½ cup sugar
1 teaspoon ground cinnamon
1 teaspoon vanilla extract
1 teaspoon maple flavoring
½ teaspoon pumpkin pie spice
½ teaspoon ground nutmeg
1 carton (8 ounces) fat-free whipped topping

In a large mixing bowl combine the cream cheese, pumpkin, and sugar substitute. Mix well. Beat in the cinnamon, vanilla, maple flavoring, pumpkin pie spice, and nutmeg. Fold in whipped topping. Refrigerate until serving.

Yield: 4 cups

Nutritional analysis: One serving (3 tablespoons) equals 33 calories, 1 g fat, 4 g carbohydrate, 1 g protein

Diabetic exchanges: ½ starch

A Diet Doc
Five Years Later

B y the time this book is released it will be five years since I walked into Joe's office. Talk about a moment that changed my life! It doesn't rank up there with my wedding day, the birth of my children, graduation from medical school, or that time I hit three home runs in one game in the eighth grade. But I know where I would have wound up if I hadn't changed my lifestyle. Surveys have shown that physicians have one of the lowest life spans—58 years!—for professionals. Many don't reach retirement, and I didn't want to end up in that statistic.

Caring for others on a daily basis is unbelievably rewarding and unbelievably draining at the same time. Fortunately I know now that it is possible to care for others *and* care for myself, although it hasn't been easy. The first few holidays after my weight loss were very difficult. Shoulder and knee injuries have slowed my training. Sometimes life is just hard and stressful. But you know what? Now I have the knowledge I need to get back on track and stay there. I don't stumble around in the dark breathing more rapidly as anxiety steadily mounts.

Am I going to fail again? Is a return to 230 pounds just around the corner? No. The fear of not knowing where to turn or what to do is gone, replaced with understanding. I am empowered and filled with gratitude for discovering this program Joe and I are sharing with you. I have benefited, my patients have benefited, and now hopefully you will benefit as well. I won't see 230, or even 200 for that matter, ever again.

I am now my own nutritionist.

I am busy living. I hope you soon will be too!

God bless,

Scott Uloth

Bibliography

Abbasi, F., et al. "High carbohydrate diets, triglyceride rich lipoproteins, and coronary heart disease risk." *American Journal of Cardiology* 85:45-48, 2000.

Acheson, K.J., et al. "Nutritional influences on lipogenesis and thermogenesis after a carbohydrate meal." *American Journal of Physiology* 246:E62-E70, 1984.

Agus, M.S.D., et al. "Dietary composition and physiologic adaptations to energy restriction." *American Journal of Clinical Nutrition* 71:901-7, 2000.

Ascherio, A., and W.C. Willet. "Health effects of transfatty acids." *American Journal of Clinical Nutrition* 66:1006S-1010S, 1997.

Atkins, R.C. *Dr. Atkins' New Diet Revolution.* New York: Avon, 2002.

Baba, N.II., et al. "High protein versus high carbohydrate hypoenergetic diet for the treatment of obese hyperinsulinemic subjects." *International Journal of Obesity* 11:1202-1206, 1999.

Brand-Miller, J.C., et al. "Glycemic index and obesity." *American Journal of Clinical Nutrition* 76:281S-285S, 2002.

Brand-Miller, J., et al. *The New Glucose Revolution.* New York: Marlowe and Company, 2003.

Bravata, D.M., L. Sanders, J. Huang, et al. "Efficacy and safety of low-carbohydrate diets: a systematic review." *Journal of the American Medical Association* 289; 14:1837-1850, 2003.

Bray, G.A. "Effect of caloric restrictions on energy expenditure in obese patients." *Lancet* 2:397-8, 1969.

————. "Low-carbohydrate diets and realities of weight loss." *Journal of the American Medical Association* 289; 14:1853-1855, 2003.

Brody, T. *Nutritional Biochemistry,* 2nd ed. San Diego: Academic Press: 1999.

Brownell, K.D., et al. "The effects of repeated cycles of weight loss and regain in rats." *Physiology Behavior* 38:459-64, 1986.

Campfield, L., F. Smith, and P. Burn. "Strategies and potential molecular targets for obesity treatment." *Science* 280:1383-1387, 1998.

Carlola, R., J.P. Harley, and C.R. Noback. *Human Anatomy and Physiology.* New York: McGraw-Hill, 1990.

Chinachoti, P. "Carbohydrates: Functionality in foods." *American Journal of Clinical Nutrition* 61:922S-929S, 1995.

Clark, L.T., K.C. Ferdinand, and D.P. Ferdinand. *Contemporary Management of the Metabolic Syndrome.* New York McMahon Publishing Group, 2003.

Crapo, P.A. "Simple versus complex carbohydrate use in the diabetic diet." *Annual Review of Nutrition* 5:95-114, 1985.

Daly, M.E., et al. "Dietary carbohydrate and insulin sensitivity: A review of the evidence and clinical implications." *American Journal of Clinical Nutrition* 66:1072-1085, 1997.

Depres, J.P., et al. "Hyperinsulinemia as an independent risk factor for ischemic heart disease." *New England Journal of Medicine* 334:952-957, 1996.

Dune, L.J. *Nutrition Almanac,* 3rd ed. New York: McGraw-Hill, 1990.

Eades, M.R., and M.D. Eades. *Protein Power.* New York: Bantam Books, 1996.

Ely, D.L. "Overview of dietary sodium effects on and interactions with cardiovascular and neuroendocrine functions." *American Journal of Clinical Nutrition* 65:594S-605S, 1997.

Erikson, R.H., and Y.S. Kim. "Digestion and absorption of dietary protein." *Annual Review of Medicine* 41:133-139, 1990.

Felig, P., et al. "Amino acid metabolism in the regulation of gluconeogenesis in man." *American Journal of Clinical Nutrition* 23:986-992, 1970.

Felig, P., J.D. Baxter, and L.A. Frohman. *Endocrinology and Metabolism,* 3rd ed. New York: McGraw-Hill, 1995.

Figlewicz, D.P., et al. "Endocrine regulation of food intake and body weight." *Journal of Laboratory and Clinical Medicine* 127:328-332, 1996.

Fisler, J.S., et al. "Nitrogen economy during very low calorie reducing diets." *American Journal of Clinical Nutrition* 35:471-486, 1982.

Flegal, K.M., et al. "Excess deaths associated with underweight, overweight, and obesity." *Journal of the American Medical Association* 293; 15:1861-68, 2005.

Ford, E.S., and S.Liu. "Glycemic index and serum high-density-lipoprotein cholesterol concentration among US adults." *Archives of Internal Medicine* 161:572-48, 2001.

Fordslund, A.H., et al. "Effect of protein intake and physical activity on twenty-four hour pattern and rate of micronutrient utilization." *American Physiology Society* E964-E976, 1999.

Foster-Powell, K., J.C. Brand-Miller, S.H.A. Holt. "International table of glycemic index and glycemic load values: 2002." *American Journal of Clinical Nutrition* 76:5-56, 2002.

Fraser, G.E., et al. "A Possible Protective Effect of Nutrition Consumption on Risk of Coronary Heart Disease—The Adventist Health Study." *Archives of Internal Medicine* 152:1416-1424, 1992.

Friedman, H.I., and B. Nylund. "Intestinal fat digestion, absorption, and transport." *American Journal of Clinical Nutrition* 33:1108-1139, 1980.

Frost, G., and A. Dornhorst. "The relevance of the glycemic index to our understanding of dietary carbohydrates." *Diabetic Medicine* 17:336-45, 2000.

Fushiki, T., et al. "Changes in glucose transporters in muscle in response to glucose." *American Journal of Physiology* 256: E580-E587, 1989.

Golay, A., et al. "Weight loss with low or high carbohydrate diet?" *International Journal of Obesity and Related Metabolic Disorders* 20:1067-1072, 1996.

Goldman, L., and J.C. Bennett. *Cecil Textbook of Medicine*, 21st ed. Philadelphia: Saunders, 2000.

Gottfried, S.S. *Biology Today.* St. Louis: Mosby, 1993.

Groff, J.L., and S.S. Gropper. *Advanced Nutrition and Human Metabolism.* Stamford, CT: Wadsworth Thomson Learning, 2000.

Gross, L.S., E.S. Ford, and S. Liu. "Increased consumption of refined carbohydrates and the epidemic of type 2 diabetes in the United States: an ecologic assessment." *American Journal of Clinical Nutrition* 79:774-9, 2004.

Holloszy, J., and W. Kohrt. "Regulation of carbohydrate and fat metabolism during and after exercise." *Annual Review of Nutrition* 16:121-138, 1996.

Holman, R.T. "George O. Burr and the discovery of essential fatty acids." *Journal of Nutrition* 118:535-540, 1988.

Hu, F.B., et al. "Adiposity as compared with physical activity in predicting mortality among women." *New England Journal of Medicine* 351:2694-703, 2004.

Hudgins, L., et al. "Relationship between carbohydrate induced hypertriglyceridemia and fatty acid synthesis in lean and obese subjects." *Journal of Lipid Research* 41:595-604, 2000.

Jenkins, D.J., et al. "Too much sugar, too much carbohydrate, or just too much?" *American Journal of Clinical Nutrition* 79:711-2, 2004.

Leaf, A., and P.C. Weber. "Cardiovascular effects of n-3 fatty acids." *New England Journal of Medicine* 318:549-557, 1988.

Leeds, A.R. "Glycemic index and heart disease." *American Journal of Clinical Nutrition* 76:286S-289S, 2002.

Leibel, R.L., M. Rosenbaum, and J. Hirsch. "Changes in energy expenditure resulting from altered body weight." *New England Journal of Medicine* 332:621-628, 1995.

Leibowitz, S.F. "Neurochemical-neuroendocrine systems in the brain controlling macronutrient intake and metabolism." *Trends in Neuroscience* 15:491-497, 1992.

Life Application Study Bible, NIV translation. Wheaton, IL: Tyndale House Publishers, 1991.

Liu, Simmin, et al. "Relation between changes in intakes in dietary fiber and grain products and changes in weight and development of obesity among middle aged women." *American Journal of Clinical Nutrition* 78:920-7, 2003.

Jacobson, M.F., and J. Hurley. *Restaurant Confidential*. New York: Workman Publishing, New York, 2002.

McArdle, W.D., F.I. Katch, and V.L. Katch. *Exercise Physiology: Energy, Nutrition, and Human Performance*, 3rd ed. Malvern, PA: Lea and Febiger, 1991.

Millward, D.J. "Metabolic demands for amino acids and the human dietary requirement." *Journal of Nutrition* 2563S-2576S, 1998.

Morris, K., et al. "Glycemic index, cardiovascular disease, and obesity." *Nutrition Reviews* 57:273-276, 1999.

Murray, M.T., and J. Beutler. *Understanding Fats and Oils*. Encinitas, CA: Progressive Health Publishing, 1996.

Nelson, J.K., et al. *Mayo Clinic Diet Manual: A Handbook of Nutrition Practices*, 7th ed. St. Louis: Mosby, 1994.

Netzer, C.T. *The Complete Book of Food Counts*. New York: Dell Publishing, 2003.

Nicholl, C.G., J.M. Polak, and S.R. Bloom. "The hormonal regulation of food intake, digestion, and absorption." *Annual Review of Nutrition* 5:213-239, 1985.

Nobels, F., et al. "Weight reduction with a high protein, low carbohydrate, caloric restricted diet: Effects on blood pressure, glucose, and insulin levels." *Netherlands Journal of Medicine* 35:295-302, 1989.

Pieke., B., et al. "Treatment of hypertriglyceridemia by two diets rich either in unsaturated fatty acids or in carbohydrates: Effects on lipoprotein subclasses, lipolytic enzymes, lipid transfer proteins, insulin, and leptin." *International Journal of Obesity* 24:1286-1296, 2000.

Pilkis, S.J., et al. "Hormonal regulation of hepatic gluconeogenesis and glycolysis." *Annual Review of Biochemistry* 57:755-783, 1988.

Rabast, U., J. Schonborn, and H. Kasper. "Dietetic treatment of obesity with low- and high-carbohydrate diets: comparative studies and clinical results." *International Journal of Obesity* 3(3):201-11, 1979.

Reed, W.D., et al. "The effects of insulin and glucagons on ketone-body turnover." *Biochemistry* 221:439-444, 1984.

Reeds, P.J., and T.W. Hutchens. "Protein requirements: From nitrogen balance to functional impact." *Journal of Nutrition* 1754S-1963-S, 1994.

Richter, E.A., T. Ploug, and H. Galbo. "Increased muscle glucose uptake after exercise." *Diabetes* 34:1041-1048, 1985.

Scriver, C.R., et al. "Normal plasma amino acid values in adults: The influence of some common physiological variables." *Metabolism* 34:868-873, 1985.

Sears, B., and B. Lawren. *Enter the Zone.* New York: Harper Collins, 1995.

Sims, E.A. "Studies in human hyperphagia." *Treatment and Management of Obesity.* New York, Harper and Row, 1974.

Souba, W.W., R.J. Smith, and D.W. Wilmore. "Glutamine Metabolism by the intestinal tract." *Journal of Parenteral Enteral Nutrition* 9:608-617, 1985.

Stewart, K.J., et al. "Exercise and Risk Factors Associated with Metabolic Syndrome in Older Adults." *American Journal of Preventative Medicine* 28(1):9-18, 2005.

Stordy, B.J., et al. "Weight gain, thermic effects of glucose and resting metabolic rate during recovery from anorexia nervosa." *American Journal of Clinical Nutrition* 30:138, 1977.

Thorne, A., and J. Wahren. "Diet-induced thermogenesis in well-trained subjects." *Clinical Physiology* 0:295-305, 1989.

Traxinger, R.R., and S. Marshall. "Role of amino acids in modulating glucose-induced desensitization of the glucose transport system." *Journal of Biological Chemistry* 264:20910-20916, 1989.

Underwood, A., and J. Adler. "Diet and genes." *Newsweek* 40-8, January 17, 2005.

Weinstein, A.R., et al. "Relationship of physical activity versus body mass index with type II diabetes in women." *Journal of the American Medical Association* 292;10:1188-9, 2004.

Wessel, T.R., et al. "Relationship of physical fitness versus body mass index with coronary artery disease and cardiovascular events in women." *Journal of the American Medical Association* 292;10:1179-87, 2004.

Westphal, S.A., M.C. Gannon, and F.Q. Nutrall. "Metabolic response to glucose ingested with various amounts of protein." *American Journal of Clinical Nutrition* 62:267-272, 1990.

Whitney, E.N., and S.R. Rolfes. *Understanding Nutrition*, 7th ed. St. Paul: West Publishing Company, 1996.

Woods, S.C., et al. "Signals that regulate food intake and energy homeostasis." *Science* 280:1378-1383, 1998.

Wolfe, B.M. "Potential role of raising dietary protein intake for reducing risk of atherosclerosis." *Canadian Journal of Cardiology* 11:127G-131G, 1995.

Yamada, T., et al. *Textbook of Gastroenterology*, 2nd ed. Philadelphia: J.B. Lippincott Company, 1995.

Young, D.B., et al. "Effects of sodium intake on steady-state potassium excretion." *American Journal of Physiology* 246:F772-F778, 1984.

Young, V.R., and J.S. Marchini. "Mechanisms and nutritional significance of metabolic responses to altered intakes of protein and amino acids, with reference to nutritional adaption in humans." *American Journal of Clinical Nutrition* 51:270-289, 1990.

About the Authors

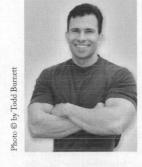

Photo © by Todd Burnett

Joe Klemczewski has degrees in physical therapy, health, and health education. In addition, he is a professional bodybuilder with an international reputation for being the nutritionist to the world's top bodybuilders and figure competitors. His website, www.thedietdoc.com, holds a wealth of nutrition and fitness information, including an active forum with members from around the world. Dr. Joe serves as a contributing science editor for Chelo Publishing in New York and writes for two of their premiere national fitness magazines *Best Body* and *Natural Bodybuilding & Fitness*. He also writes for eDiets.com and maturemensfitness.com.

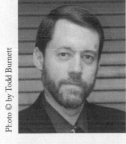

Photo © by Todd Burnett

J. Scott Uloth is a board-certified family medicine specialist, a member of the American Society of Bariatric Physicians, and is certified by the American Board of Geriatrics. Scott maintains a medical practice in Southern Indiana. He is also a clinical instructor for the Indiana University School of Medicine and received teaching awards in 1995 and 2002 from the American Academy of Teachers of Family Practice and the American Academy of Family Physicians respectively.

For more information on health, fitness, and
the Diet Docs' Rx, visit www.thedietdoc.com

Other Excellent Books on Health from Harvest House Publishers

Overcoming Back and Neck Pain

Lisa Morrone

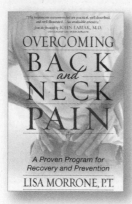

One third of Americans report having low-back pain in the last 30 days. Ten percent are enduring chronic neck pain right now. Are you one of them? If so, you know that drug prescriptions, endless treatments, and limited lifestyles are some of the consequences.

Expert physical therapist Lisa Morrone helps you say no to the treadmill of suffering. From nearly 20 years of teaching and practicing physical therapy, she offers a proven approach to overcoming nagging back and neck pain.

Lisa puts in one straightforward, accessible package the most effective exercises, guidelines, and lifestyle adjustments, involving...

- proper posture and core stability
- strengthening and stretching
- healthy movement patterns and ergonomics
- recovery from pain from compressed or ruptured discs
- nutrition, rest, and emotional/spiritual issues

Following Lisa's recommendations, you can attain substantial or complete freedom from pain. Experience the freedom to enjoy work, friends, family, and fulfilling service to God again!

Overcoming Headaches and Migraines
Lisa Morrone

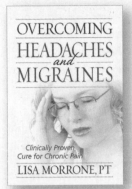

In this comprehensive, multifaceted resource, physical therapist Lisa Morrone gives you clear help and practical guidelines for overcoming or eliminating migraines. You can achieve lasting changes by uncovering head–pain sources, such as neck or muscle problems; starting new habits and exercises; avoiding migraine and cluster headache triggers; and tackling stress, anger, and emotional/spiritual bondage.

Overcoming Runaway Blood Sugar
Dennis Pollock

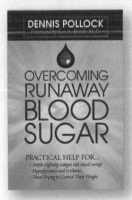

After author Dennis Pollock experienced a serious diabetic episode, his desire to understand the whys of blood sugar fluctuation, its potential damage to the body, and the ways of prevention led him on a quest for answers. Now Pollock helps you achieve optimum health by exploring

- what you should know about the blood sugar delivery system

- reasons to change your lifestyle and why faith is a great motivator

- a diet and exercise program that works

Good health comes when good information is followed by action. Dennis will help you trade fatigue, weight gain, and illness brought on by unhealthy blood sugar levels for a life of optimum health.

BASIC Steps to Godly Fitness
Laurette Willis

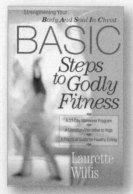

In this uniquely integrated program, certified personal trainer and aerobics instructor Laurette Willis shares her BASIC (Body And Soul In Christ), step-by-step plan to improve wholeness in your body, soul, and spirit.

Laurette gives you plenty of practical opportunities for growth, including "PraiseMoves," her unique Christian system of worship and exercise she calls "a Christ-centered alternative to yoga."

Praise Moves DVD
Laurette Willis

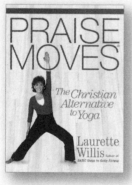

For 22 years Laurette Willis studied yoga and endured a difficult journey through New Age beliefs. When she became a Christian, she was given the desire to create a Christian alternative to yoga. Now churches across America host her PraiseMoves program. With this DVD you can...

• increase your flexibility and balance

• lose weight and gain endurance

• nurture a rich, meaningful prayer life

• ease depression and stress and inspire joy

With two workouts—60 and 20 minutes each—that are easy, effective, and intended for all fitness levels, you can get started right away.

Make your exercise time one of worshiping God and achieving health and rejuvenation.